Napiers'
VEGETABLE LAXATIVE TABLETS
For Constipation and Sluggish Liver

DOSE—One or two tablets at bedtime, or one night and morning.

Each tablet contains—Ex. Colon. Co. 1 gr.; Rx. Jalap. 1 gr.; Rx. Taras. 1 gr.; Rx. Podoph. 1 gr.; Leptandrin 1 gr.; Ol. Menth. Pip.q.s.

D. NAPIER & SONS
17-18 Bristo Place, EDINBURGH.1

Napiers'
PRUNIN HEART TONIC

This Tonic has a direct influence over the Heart and the digestive apparatus, and a simultaneous sedative action on the nerves and circulation. For Palpitation, altering irritability and giving a natural sleep, the Heart Tonic removes that feeling of debility brought on through ill health, overwork or anxiety. It restores the appetite for food and brings fresh blood, thus giving new life to the Heart. As the Tonic acts the Heart gains strength, the flow of blood becomes fuller, the feet and hands lose their coldness, the nerve headaches begin to leave, pains disappear, then comes the sensation of renewed health and growing strength.

Directions: SHAKE THE BOTTLE, and take from 20-30 drops in a little water, four times daily after food.

Compounded from; 40% Alcoholic tincture. Scullcap (1 in 5) 4; Skunk Cabbage (1 in 5) 4 drs.; Crawci (1 in 5) 4 drs.; Cayenne (1 in 7) 1 dr.; American Valerian BHP 0.76 ml; Cactus (1 in 5) 4.75; Pulsatilla (1 in 5) 4.5; Motherwort (1 pt 4); 5; Lily of the Valley (1 in 5) 4.5; Hawthorn Berries (1 in 4) 4.5; 45%; Alcoholic Extract Wild Cherry Bark B.P.C. (1 in 5) and 100%; PRICE (including Tax) 3/-

D. NAPIER & SONS
BRITISH AND FOREIGN MEDICAL BOTANISTS
17-18 Bristo Place, EDINBURGH, 1

Napiers
ROSEMARY HAIR TONIC

for correction of greasiness and prevention of dandruff & for greying hair

Massage briskly but gently into the hair and scalp, 2 or 3 times a week, followed by a good brushing

Compounded from:
Aqueous extract of Rosemary 5; Oil of Basin Geranium 0.1; Oil of Cedarwood 0.1; Oil of Lemon 0.1

D. NAPIER & SONS
British and Foreign
Medical Botanists
17-18 Bristo Place
EDINBURGH, 1

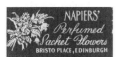

NAPIERS'
Perfumed Sachet Flowers
BRISTO PLACE, EDINBURGH

Herbal
Tonic Tablets
PL 0896/5023

Dose : Two Tablets three times daily
Ex. Damiana 16.2 mg; Ex Saw Palmetto 16.2 mg; Skullcap 16.2 mg; Convallaria 16.2 mg. (BPC 1949)

D. NAPIER & SONS
British and Foreign Medical Botanists
17-18 Bristo Place, EDINBURGH, 1

P.L 0896/5002
NAPIERS' HERBAL OINTMENT
RED
...the Skin

D0871981

NAPIERS' HERBAL POWDER
COMPOUND COMFREY

To help relieve the discomfort of haemorrhoids and discourage bleeding by softening the stool

Dose.—A rounded teaspoonful. Place the dose in a teacup, fill with boiling water and mix thoroughly. Drink the clear liquid when doses should be taken daily, the first after breakfast, the time. A dose may be prepared at night so as to be ready 1g. Each dose should be made separately.

ingredient:—Each rounded teaspoonful contains approx:
g; Bistort 0.25 g; Rhubarb 0.25 g; Barberry 0.25 g; g; Am. Cranesbill 0.1 g; Ginger 0.1 g; Mountain Grape cal 0.04 g; Stone Root 0.1 g; Yarrow 0.1 g; Blue Flag

MEDICINES OUT OF REACH OF CHILDREN
PL 0896/5041
D. NAPIER & SONS
17/18 Bristo Place, EDINBURGH

NAPIERS'
TONIC BLOOD PURIFIER

For use in cases of skin irritation and other minor skin conditions
Dose.—1 of a 5 ml teaspoonful in a wineglass of water, three or four times daily after meals.

Active Ingredients—Each 5 ml contains; 25% Alcohol Ext. 3 of Lappa BHP 0.135 ml; Trifolium BHP 0.135 ml; Burdr. Aquif. Angostura BHP 0.135 ml; Rumex Crispus 0.135 ml 40%; Alcohol Ext. of Phytolacca BHP 0.135 ml; 45%; Alcohol Zanthoxylum BHP 0.06 ml
(1 in 5) Tinct. 45%; Alcohol. Acaia BHP 0.06 ml; Scutellaria 0.135 ml; Tinct. Capsicum BPC 1968 0.06 ml; Tinct. Cimicifuga BPC 1934 0.06 ml; Tinct. Valerian BPC 1949 0.06 ml; Inf. Calumba BPC 0.135 ml.

KEEP MEDICINES OUT OF REACH OF CHILDREN
SHAKE THE BOTTLE
PL 0896/502
D. NAPIER & SONS
17/18 Bristo Place, EDINBURGH

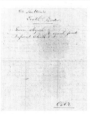

Preserve this Card and return for a renewal of Medicine

ESTABLISHED 1860

D. NAPIER & SONS
JOHN R. NAPIER,
Consultant Member of the British Herbalist's Union

British and Foreign Medical Botanists & Consulting Herbalists

17 & 18 BRISTO PLACE
EDINBURGH

TELEPHONE · · · CENtral 5542

NAPIERS'
S and CALENDULA

Rub into the parts with the finger, gently but firmly, 1, 2 or 3 times daily.

Prepared from—Calendula 1 3, Sambutus 3, Trifolium 5, Alkanet 5, Ulmus Fulva 1 25, Cera Alb. 2 75, Spermaceti 25, Acid Salph 1, Adeps 13, Sapit. Soft. 95, Paraffin dur. 15, Paraff. Moll. (If Ol. Rapit 16, Cetaceum 1 5.

D. NAPIER & SONS
British & Foreign Medical Botanists
15, 17 & 18 BRISTO PLACE
EDINBURGH, 1

NAPIER'S
Nerve Debility Tonic
To restore perfect health to the nerves.

The Compound of Nerve Tonics rebuilds the nervous power; restores debility to health, and gives new life to the nerves. This nerve to health remedy through the entire nervous system, directs all nerve weaknesses nourishly taken. Under the curative effect of the Tonic the appetite returns, digestion improves, and the blood becomes richer. With the return of nerve health, nervous headache, insomnia and despondency vanish. The headaches become natural and refreshing, then life asserts itself with new energy to carry on the pleasant sensation of perfect health.

DOSE—20 to 30 drops in a wine glassful of water four times daily after meals and at bedtime. SHAKE THE BOTTLE.
To relieve of Tea and Coffee, take More sand Dandelion Coffee and use pure Nippony Kyo Hock as additional food.
PRICE (including tax) 3/18.

FORMULA: 30% Alcoholic Extracts (1-1); Scullcap 7.5; Convallaria 7.5; Kola 7.5; Damiana 7.5; Euonymus 7.5; Rhuem 1.5; 35% Alcoholic Extract (1-2.5; Calumba 2, 80%; Alcoholic Tinctures of Hops (1 in 5); Capsicum (1-7); 45%; Alcoholic Tinctures of Steam Celandine 3.5; Pancretis (1-4); American Rootwood (1-10)4; Cramps (1-14); Glycerine (to 100%).

D. NAPIER & SONS
British and Foreign Medical Botanists
17-18 Bristo Place, EDINBURGH, 1

FOR EXTERNAL USE ONLY
NAPIERS'
SASSAFRAS
FOR
UNBROKEN CHILBLAINS

Directions — Rub the LINIMENT into the Chilblains thoroughly but gently with cotton wool, if very tender paint with a camel hair brush. This should be done at night and the Chilblains covered with flannel or soft white lint. Repeat the application twice or three times during the day. The affected parts should not be held near the fire nor rubbed with cold winds.

Compounded from the following;—Curcuma 2.75, Sassafras 2.75, Ammon. Carb. 2.75, Capsicum 3.5, Liq. Anthron. Fort 1.25, Ol. Tornbtenth. 10, Soy. Vin. Meth. (In.lutl.) to produce 100, Ol. Camph. Terpol. 100.

D. NAPIER & SONS
BRITISH AND FOREIGN MEDICAL BOTANISTS
17-18 Bristo Place, EDINBURGH, 1

Napiers
Tonic
Shampoo

D. NAPIER & SON
BRISTO PLACE
EDINBURGH

PL 0896/5005
NAPIERS' HERBAL OINTMENT
Poke Root

For the relief of hard skin, dry, scaly, itchy patches, eczema, and psoriasis.

Directions:—Rub into the parts with the fingers, thoroughly but gently 2 or 3 times daily; or apply on gauze 2 or 3 times daily.

Active Ingredients:—Extract of (Trifol. 2; Symphytum 2; Calendula 2; Ulmus Fulv. 2; Phyrolac.4) in (Paraff. Dur 25; Paraff. Mol 25; Ol. Cocois 8; Ol. Rapii 22; Ol. Arachis 8) 100%.

Keep medicines out of reach of children
D. NAPIER & SONS
17/18 BRISTO PLACE
EDINBURGH

NAPIERS'
NASAL CATARRH MIXTURE

For Nasal Catarrh, the result of neglected colds, fullness of head, and loss of taste and smell.

Dose.—1 of a 5 ml teaspoonful in a wineglass of water, three or four times daily—taken in sips, gargled and swallowed.

Active Ingredients. Each 15 ml contains,—Tinct. Sanguinaria BHP 0.5 ml; Tinct. Capsicum BPC 1968 0.03 ml; Tinct. Symplocarpus BHP 0.03 ml; Tinct. Scutellaria BHP 0.06 ml; Tinct. Valerian BPC 1949 0.025 ml; Tinct. Cimicifuga BPC 1934 0.037 ml; Tinct. Hydrastis RPC 1949 0.037 ml; Tinct. Lobelia BPC 1949 0.012 ml; Liq. Ext. Viburnum Op. BHP 0.017 ml; Liq. Ext. Herb. Aquif BHP 0.037 ml.

KEEP MEDICINES OUT OF REACH OF CHILDREN
SHAKE THE BOTTLE
PL 0896/5019
D. NAPIER & SONS,
17/18 Bristo Place, Edinburgh

NAPIERS'
No. 2 Lotion

For rashes and minor skin conditions.
For use where ointments are not practical.
For external use only

Directions—Rub into the parts gently two or three times daily.
Active Ingredients.—Tinc. Benz. Simp. BPC 2%; (1 in 5) 25%; Alcohol Ext. Rubus Id. 2%; Tinc. Calendula BPC 1934 2%; Tinc. Barthisia BPC 1934 2%.
KEEP MEDICINES OUT OF REACH OF CHILDREN
SHAKE THE BOTTLE
PL 0896/5058
D. NAPIER & SONS
17 & 18 BRISTO PLACE
EDINBURGH. 1

Napier's
HERB SMOKING MIXTURE

The "BRISTO BRAND" has been used for nearly a century by those wishing a pleasant, fragrant and agreeable smoke, and one which can do no hurt to nerves, digestion or heart. The rare combination of leaves and flowers produces a unique meaning of pleasure, giving soothing relief and satisfaction of the Perfect Smoke. Inhaled, the smoke is relaxant and balsamic, helping to dislodge phlegm and clear choked breathing tubes.

Formula : Althaea 30, Tussilago 30, Rubus 28, Trifolium 4, Lavand 8.

D. NAPIER & SONS
BRITISH & FOREIGN MEDICAL BOTANISTS
17 and 18 BRISTO PLACE, EDINBURGH, 1.

PULMONARY LOZENGES

D. NAPIER & SONS
17 & 18 BRISTO PLACE
EDINBURGH, 1

NAPIERS'
SOOTHING SYRUP
FOR INFANTS

A herbal remedy for stomach disorders in children including those due to teething.

Dose.— (1) For babies under 6 months: 10 drops (2) For babies 6-18 months; 15 drops (3) For children over 18 months: One 5 ml teaspoonful. In each case to be given in a little warm water, night and morning.

Active Ingredients.—Each 10 drops contains approx. The Aqu. Ext. from Balm 20 mg; Rhubarb 20 mg; Aniseed 20 mg; Senna 20 mg; Elder 10 mg; Pennyroyal 5 mg.
Each 5 ml spoonful contains approx. The Aqu. Ext. from Balm 0.1 g; Rhubarb 0.1 g; Aniseed 0.1 g; Senna 0.1 g; Elder 0.05 g; Pennyroyal 0.025 g.
KEEP MEDICINES OUT OF REACH OF CHILDREN
SHAKE THE BOTTLE
PL 0896/5013
D. NAPIER & SONS
17/18 BRISTO PLACE, EDINBURGH

Napiers
History of Herbal Healing,
Ancient and Modern

TOM ATKINSON

Napiers
History of Herbal Healing,
Ancient and Modern

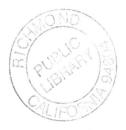

TOM ATKINSON

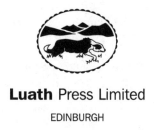

Luath Press Limited

EDINBURGH

www.luath.co.uk

First published 2003

The paper used in this book is recyclable. It is made from low
chlorine pulps produced in a low energy, low emission manner
from renewable forests.

Printed and bound by
Cromwell Press, Trowbridge

Typeset in 10.5 Sabon by
S Fairgrieve, Edinburgh, 0131 658 1763

Contents

Foreword

IN 1860, DUNCAN SCOTT NAPIER opened a herb shop and a part-time herbalist practice in Bristo Place, Edinburgh. Duncan was a young man, a baker by trade, and newly married. He was also, in the old Scots expression, a 'bastard wean', who had been adopted as an infant by the Napier family. They kept an inn on the outskirts of Edinburgh.

It is difficult to understand why the Napiers adopted the baby. They certainly showed no love for him. Both alcoholics, the husband, although not himself ill-treating the child, did nothing to prevent the wife from doing so, and Duncan suffered much from her, as he describes in an autobiography he drafted much later.

A miserably unhappy childhood, with little education – this was long before the days of compulsory education – led to a youth of hard work as an apprentice baker. One early morning, while on his daily round of delivering new-baked rolls, he was accosted by Mr John Hope, a gentleman (and the term is surely well justified), who habitually took his daily walk on the same road.

After many early morning conversations, John Hope had a profound effect on Duncan, who was encouraged to seek further education, to foreswear alcohol, and to become a convinced Christian. As time passed, Mr Hope also helped Duncan in many material ways.

Somehow, Duncan developed an interest in gardening, and out of that, an interest in herbs and their healing powers. At this stage entirely self-taught by reading everything he could find about herbs, he rapidly acquired a considerable knowledge not only of herbs and their properties, but also of the human body, its ailments and the effect of herbs on illness.

He treated himself, his family and his workmates, and eventually had the tremendous self-confidence to open a herb shop and part-time herbalist practice in Bristo Place, Edinburgh, a street then bordering on some of the worst slums in the city.

Clearly, there was a considerable demand for a herbalist in

mid-Victorian Edinburgh, and the business and practice grew rapidly, so much so that Duncan gave up the baking trade and became a full-time herbalist.

Duncan was followed into the business by two sons and a grandson, each of whom, more formally trained and educated than Duncan, continued the tradition of herbal healing which he established. Moreover, they did a great deal to place the business on a sound footing, not just financial, but also scientific. Duncan himself had flourished well enough financially, and grew from being the unhappy lad who never had a penny to spend, and whose clothes were invariably patched and well-worn, to the status of being well established in the middle class, and able to ensure that his sons were well educated.

John Napier, the last of his line, died suddenly in 1978, and his widow, who was not a qualified herbalist, did her best to continue the practice and business, being greatly helped by her family and qualified friends.

Gradually, though, the business and practice declined, until, in 1992, it was taken over by a newly qualified, dynamic young herbalist. Rapid expansion and development followed.

To understand why herbal medicine flourishes today, it is essential to know something of its long history, from its origins in the dim dawn-light of humanity's appearance on this earth, to its present position as the major, often the only, source of skilled medical help for the majority of people in the world. Furthermore, even in those societies where conventional medical help is available, like our own, herbalism continues to be in great demand as a therapy complementary to that of the allopathic, or conventional, doctor.

Since this book is mainly concerned with one particular herbal establishment in Scotland, the main emphasis is on herbalism and its practise in that country. But it tells also of herbalism in its world-wide context. The healing herbs used in Scotland were those which grew there: the English herbalists used their local herbs, and so did those in America, in Canada and virtually every other country. But that was long ago, and the herbalist of today has access to herbs from every part of the world.

Furthermore, not only does the trained herbalist of today use herbs from many countries, she also has knowledge of the healing skills of other traditions from many sources.

Furthermore again, she has access to the scientific evaluation and testing of those many herbs and their uses. A modern herbalist is an holistic healer in the true sense of the word. It is not symptoms that are treated, but the whole being.

After looking at the long history of herbal medicine world-wide, this book centres on Scotland, especially the Highlands, and describes many of the herbal treatments once the only form of medicine available. Then, after reviewing the society in which Duncan Napier lived and worked in mid-Victorian Scotland, the book moves on to Duncan Napier himself. As an Appendix, there is an unfinished and unpublished autobiography by Duncan. This rather sad hand-written document describes his strange upbringing by a sadistic step-mother, his burgeoning interest in herbs and healing, the opening of his shop and some cases he dealt with – and cured. The document ends abruptly when Duncan was describing how two of his sons died as the result of the newly com-pulsory vaccination against smallpox.

Two of Duncan's sons followed him into the business and herbal practice. Both well-educated, and with a sound scientific training, they guided the growing business through many traumas and problems. The last of the Napier family to practise herbalism was Duncan's grandson, John, who died untimely in 1978. Between them they saw the business through two world wars (in which they played a gallant part), and repeated attempts by Government to outlaw the practice of herbalism and the use of herbs for healing.

After a period of decline following John Napier's death, the business was eventually taken over by a young, professionally trained and energetic young woman herbalist. Still with its head-quarters in Duncan's original premises in Edinburgh, there are now two branches in Edinburgh, one in Glasgow, two in London, one in Chichester and one in Bristol. Others are imminent.

The book ends with a survey of herbalism in Britain today, and its continued precarious position under frequent attack by Govern-ment and the massed ranks of the medical and pharmaceutical professions. There is also an account by a young Scottish herbalist of today of how she was trained and educated in her profession, and of how the apprenticeship system of training is still followed by Napiers of Edinburgh.

Still based on the solid foundations laid down by the Napier family, the business is heading confidently into the 21st century, utilising every possible modern resource, whilst retaining all the ethics, the warmth and the humanity and charity of traditional healing. It is, in fact, a social history of an essential and neglected part of our national heritage.

Introduction

An inconsiderable planet, a speck in the infinite stellar wastes; most of it salt water, the bulk of the land rock and desert and austral and boreal ice, interspersed mud, the detritus of aeons, with a thin coverlet of grass and trees – that vegetable world on which every living thing was in the last resort a parasite!

John Buchan *Sick Heart River*

BOTTLES OF MEDICINE. Probably every household in the country has them. They stand in innumerable cupboards, bathroom cabinets and kitchen dressers, often dusty and forgotten, with a stained label stating 'Two tablespoonsful to be taken in water three times a day after meals', or something like that.

Those old neglected bottles lurking in unexpected places are a symbol of mankind's perennial hope that somewhere there is a cure for his ills. This faith in health-giving drugs is as old as humanity itself. I have long wondered why it is always three times a day, and not twice or four times. Perhaps it is because three is a magic number, a sacred triad in many societies, as the Trinity in Christianity, as Brahma, Vishnu and Shiva, the three gods of Hinduism responsible for the creation of the universe, and in the even more ancient Sankhya philosophy as the three gunas or creative forces, the ragas, tamas and sattva.

In the Zagros mountains of north-east Iraq there are many caves. The people of the area, at least until very recently, were semi-nomadic Kurds, who used the caves for shelter, and, they said, had always done so.

Such folk memories are often useful guidance for archaeologists. If local people said a site or cave had 'always' been used, it is probably worth a dig. The archaeologist Ralph Solecki certainly thought so, and in 1951 began investigating the Zagros caves.

Preliminary digs in various places produced nothing of much interest, but after a month or so, Solecki asked the local people for advice. He was told of the Big Cave of Shanidor, which was still used every year as shelter. When Solecki located Shanidor, he found what he said was the most magnificent cave he had ever seen – truly a big cave, the south-facing entrance meant that the sun gave light and heat, kept the floor dry, and generally provided an ideal dwelling and shelter from bad weather and heat. If the Kurds were still using this ideal place, perhaps their ancestors had indeed 'always' used it. And if they had used it, then they surely had left traces.

The dig began in the autumn, after the nomadic Kurds had moved on. Five feet down into the earth floor, the archaeologists began to find interesting material. It was not dramatic stuff, merely stone chippings and charred wood, and was dated as being no more than 10,000 years old. But it was an encouraging beginning, and if 10,000 years was not really 'always', perhaps there was more to discover still deeper.

Two years later, Solecki and a much larger team returned. Soon they came upon the first really exciting find, the remains of a Neanderthal infant. This was indeed important, for the remains were dated as being about 60,000 years old. Clearly, humans and their ancestors had used this cave over aeons of time.

If there were the remains of one Neanderthal there, the probability was there would be others, perhaps even the remains of the parents of that infant. Further digging, in 1957, revealed three adult males. Before the dig was completed, two more adult males were found, together with two adult females and another infant, nine remains in all.

Each of those remains was important, and each added something to our knowledge of the Neanderthal people, one of our distant ancestors. Three of the males had died several thousand years after the others. All had been buried with care, and, it appeared, with some ceremony. Two of the later group had been disabled for some years before their death, and this discovery was itself important. It meant that the Neanderthals had cared for those disabled people for years, and thus were not the uncaring, brutal characters they had been branded.

However, much the most important find was connected with

the fourth remains found, known still as Shanidor 4. There was nothing particularly remarkable about the remains themselves, except their age, of course. It was the soil around those remains that carried the most important discovery of all.

A skeleton, given the right conditions, will last for an eternity of years, and skilled examination can tell us much about the life, illnesses, injuries and death of that person. The pollen of plants, in the right conditions, is equally long lasting, and perhaps even more informative.

Not only does each type of pollen tell us of the plant from which it came, it can tell us of the season and the climate. Paleobotanical examination of the soil around Shanidor 4 showed pollen from 28 species of plants. Of that 28, seven were grouped in clusters which seemed to have been woven into the twigs of a pine-like shrub.

It appeared that Shanidor 4 man had been buried, or laid to rest, accompanied by a carefully woven wreath. But there was more to be learned from the pollen of the funeral wreath. The plants were hollyhock, yarrow, groundsel, St. Barnaby's thistle, cornflower, marshmallow and grape hyacinth. The seventh plant, which did not form part of the wreath, was strewn deeply under the bones, as though to form a bed, a last resting place for this man. That plant was yarrow, whose springy woody stem is still used by the Kurds as beds.

That was astonishing enough. What is even more astonishing is that, apart from hollyhock, each and every one of those plants has a powerful medicinal action, and every one is still used today, 60,000 years later, in the practice of herbal medicine.

Those plants are still used by the local people of Iraq as well as being used by herbalists world-wide. The roots of marshmallow soothe sore throats and ease digestive problems, and the leaves are for the lungs and urinary system. Grape hyacinth is a diuretic and a digestive stimulant. Yarrow, an astringent, is also an insect repellent and general tonic. Groundsel is, amongst other things, a purgative and useful in the treatment of intestinal worms. The thistle is used for the relief of kidney and bladder stones, and for gravel. Cornflower, often used to soothe eyes, is a general tonic and stimulant and also an emmenagogue, a uterine tonic and a stimulant for menstrual flow.

Was that Neanderthal man we know as Shanidor 4 a healer who used those herbs to treat his fellows? Or perhaps the wreath was made up of healing plants to ease his passage to somewhere different? We can never know that.

I find it particularly moving that hollyhock was included in the wreath. As a close relative of marshmallow, hollyhock does have some value as a soothing digestive herb, although not much. However, hollyhock is a plant that in the wild does not grow in clumps or beds. The plants always grow alone, and often far apart. Someone, 60,000 years ago, wandered widely over the hills, gathering those hollyhocks and weaving them into the carefully prepared wreath. That is not the act of some savage brute of a caveman: rather it indicates care and thought, even love.

That Big Cave of Shanidor has provided us with the earliest record, so far, of using plants for healing. For much, indeed for the vast majority, of human history, there are no written records. We must rely on the evidence of archaeology for our knowledge of those many centuries, and that evidence is inevitably patchy, found by chance, and always open to interpretation and question. Only when written records appear, and only when those records can be interpreted, can we speak with certainty of the knowledge and practices of our ancestors.

Even before the discovery of writing, some ancient societies left records of their healers. There is, for example, the Cave of the Three Brothers in the Pyrenees. On a wall of that great cave, which was a prehistoric dwelling for many centuries, there is a vivid painting of a healer. He – and it is unmistakably a male – is dressed in the skin of an animal, and his limbs are striped with alternate bands of light and dark paint. A set of deer antlers is fastened to his head, and he appears to be treating a patient lying prone before him. There is no indication of what treatment that ancient healer is using, but it was probably some ritual or ceremony. Interestingly, many thousands of years later, the antlered stag was adopted by Christianity as the symbol for Christ's struggle against evil, and it is reasonable to suppose a direct connection between that ancient healer painted so graphically on the cave wall and the symbol chosen to represent struggle against evil, or illness.

The earliest written records of herbal medicine of which we know at present come from China. In 2800 BC, a herbalist called Shen Nung wrote his Pen Ts'ao. This describes treatments for many illnesses, but also lists and describes no less than 364 plants Shen Nung used in his treatments. Most of them are still in use today.

From then on, there has been a steady stream of writings about herbs and herbal medicine. Every known civilisation which has developed a form of writing has used that writing to record the use of herbs in healing.

The story, the romance, of herbal medicine has been well recorded. What is not so familiar is the actual story of those who have practised herbal medicine in the recent past, and continue to do so today.

This book is the story of Napiers of Edinburgh, established in 1860, one of the last herbal houses in Britain where herbalism is practised, and, under one roof, herbal products are produced, herbal prescriptions dispensed, herbal students trained, and herbal research conducted.

It is a fascinating story and an important record. It happens that I am the father of Dee Atkinson, a consulting herbalist at Napiers, and one of the present owners of the business. She is the first person to be in that position and yet not be a member of the Napier family. She tells me that she feels herself to be the descendant not only of Duncan Napier, the founder of the practice and shop, but of all the countless herbalists and healers who have gone before, enriching us with their knowledge and their experience. She is sure that she would have much to discuss with Shen Nung if only it was possible to be transported back through time for 5,000 years. And although it would be difficult to communicate, I, like her, would dearly love to ask that distant ancestor of ours why, 60,000 years ago, he or she felt impelled to wander over the hills seeking hollyhocks to weave into a wreath for a man newly dead.

PART I

Herbalism through the Ages

He causeth the grass to grow for the cattle and herbs for the service of man.

Psalm 104.2

BEFORE FOCUSSING ON SCOTTISH HERBALISM, and specifically on Napiers of Edinburgh, we should determine just what herbalism and herbal medicine really are.

Perhaps massage is the oldest form of treatmenta still in use today. It seems to be an instinctive thing for us to rub ourselves to ease the pains of a fall or a blow, and massage is maybe a sophisticated way of doing that. However, herbalism is certainly the oldest form of medicine, if not perhaps of treatment. Simply, it is the use of plant remedies in the treatment of disease. Not only is it the oldest known form of medicine, it is still the most widely used, world-wide. We have all noticed how our domesticated dogs and cats will instinctively eat plants, usually grass, if they feel unwell, and I have frequently watched a rather lazy old Jersey cow, a great family favourite, get up from her rest under a shady tree and walk a hundred yards to where a favourite herb grew, snatch a few mouthfuls, and immediately return to her resting place, her quiet cud-chewing and perhaps her contemplation of the world. I am sure that that particular herb – it was young meadow-sweet – soothed a passing discomfort in one of her stomachs, just as a herbalist will use meadowsweet today. Very possibly a similar instinct impelled our very distant ancestors to try eating certain plants if they were ill. Gradually, over untold generations, a con-siderable body of knowledge was acquired about the healing or soothing powers of certain plants.

Remember, we are not speaking about a few thousand years, but speaking rather of hundreds of thousands, going way back into the first glimmering of dawn light in the history of humans and humanoids.

As those ancient peoples spread, out of Africa probably, so the knowledge of healing with herbs spread with them, for of course there was no alternative method of healing. In each area, as those ancient peoples occupied and colonised, there were new plants to try and evaluate. India, China, the myriad islands dotting what today we call the Pacific Ocean, the vast continent of the Americas, the varied immensity of Europe – all provided potential new plant material for trial and, no doubt, error.

Somehow, in those distant days long before the invention of writing, some individuals acquired the reputation of being skilled in treating illnesses. Perhaps they just had a natural curiosity about the mysteries of illness and healing and death. Perhaps they had particularly good memories, so that they could recall the effects that using different herbs would have, just as others had memories enabling them to hunt and to lead hunts, and others to remember the ancestry of the group, its songs and rituals.

One historian of today has described the hunter-gatherer period of human history as 'the longest clinical trial in history, which eventually produced the herbs that provided the best foods, the poisons to destroy enemies, the finest fuels and weapons, soporific drinks, medicines, the plants that produce colours for body and cave painting, and the 'magic' plants that carried primitive man away from reality.'

It is the few remote tribespeople who still live in jungle, forest, desert or marshland who can provide the most information about the primitive medicine of our common ancestors. Almost every tribe of people, wherever it lives and whatever its degree of sophistication, has its men or women priests, its medical men or medicine women. Today, as outsiders, we can study the beliefs and practices of those 'primitive' peoples, although it is very unlikely that even the most friendly and sympathetic of observers will ever be shown or told the true secrets of the healer. These, generally, are passed on from the medicine man or woman, the repository of medical knowledge, to a successor who is trained and trusted. This secrecy, the determination to keep to themselves the innermost secrets of healing, is why few western observers have ever been able to gain more than a superficial knowledge of what is in fact frequently a highly developed system of healing, both mental and physical, amongst peoples still regarded as primitive.

We do know that each people slowly built up a herbal *materia medica* based on the local plant life. Obviously, there must have been much experimentation, and indeed many errors. However, perhaps the errors were limited because so many of the plants we know to be harmful or poisonous are themselves unattractive, like the familiar deadly nightshade, or else give early warning by being highly irritant, like hemlock or spurge.

The careful observation and experiments with plants must have gone on for thousands of years, with the medicine man or woman carefully noting which part of the plant is most active – leaf, flower, root, stem, bark or fruit – and when in its growing season it was most active and potent. How was it most effectively administered? As a poultice or as an infusion, or perhaps best simmered in water? Over those thousands of years, a very great body of empirical knowledge was acquired, passed down through the many generations of healers, and, eventually, written down when that particular tribe or civilisation acquired the skill of writing.

Doctors and pharmacists have always scorned the idea that the powers, healing or harmful, of plants could vary with the time of day or phase of the moon, or the season. And yet, time and again, it has been shown that the alkaloid type and content of plants does indeed vary with the clock and the season and the moon, and it is this alkaloid quality that gives many plants their potency and medicinal action. That knowledge, and the act of harvesting accordingly, was established by comparatively primitive peoples long ago: it is followed today by those who carefully harvest herbs for their medicinal action.

It was only when the ancient hunter-gatherer peoples developed into agriculturists that settled communities and eventually cities appeared. It became possible for specialisation of labour to be followed, and for the trading of labour to begin. One man became a skilled carpenter, his neighbour skilled at growing crops. It was an obvious step for the carpenter to build a hut for his crop-growing neighbour, who in return 'paid' for the labour with his grain or roots. Out of such simplicity there arose the complexity of the city life we know today, with all its specialisations, including, of course, that of healing, as well as that of writing about healing. It was when the ancient form of human or humanoid social organisation had developed into settled communities that the strange art and skill of writing appeared, and amongst the very first things written were accounts of the plants used in healing, and of how they were to be used.

Obviously, the healer's knowledge was held in great respect: it had therefore to be recorded for all time to come, along with the history of the people, and the genealogies of the leading members of the community, the kings and warriors.

But in some societies, Babylon for instance, it was believed that skill in healing was not confined to the professional healer, but was known to all people, as part of their common heritage. Herodotus tells us that the people of Babylon were so interested in disease and its treatment that they laid their sick people out in the streets of the city in order that passers-by could give advice:

> They bring out their sick in the market place, for they have no physicians; then those who pass by the sick person confer with him about the disease to discover whether they themselves have been afflicted with the same disease as the sick person, or have seen others so afflicted; then the passers-by talk to him and advise him to have recourse to the same treatment as that by which they have escaped a similar disease or as they have known to cure others. And they are not allowed to pass by a sick person in silence without enquiring the nature of the distemper.

It was a situation perhaps not so very unlike that of today, when our friends and colleagues and family happily advise us of their successful cures when we happen to catch whatever is 'going around' at present.

As time passed, the centuries and generations saw the once isolated communities and civilisations begin trading with each other, and amongst the goods traded were vast quantities of herbs and plants. Amongst the cargo of that '*Quinquireme of Ninevah, from distant Ophir, rowing home to haven in sunny Palestine*', there would certainly be the sandalwood and cedarwood and sweet white wine of the poem, but there would also be bales of castor oil seeds, of linseed and of dried white poppies for opium. There would be small packages of cannabis, used as a sedative and painkiller, saffron, and perhaps garlic, juniper and fennel, all used for the treatment of illness by the healers, the doctors.

Although several herbal books of that period at about the beginning of the Christian era have survived, none of them is of particular note, nor are they innovations, except for one, and of that only fragments survive. This was the work of Crataeus, physician to Mithradates VI, King of Pantus. The King was himself, it seems, a dabbler in medicine, and at his suggestion Crataeus wrote a 'herbal', and for the first time illustrated it with 'painted likenesses of plants', together with a description of their virtues and uses. This became the pattern or template for all subsequent books about herbs and their uses in healing, and we still, more than 2,000 years later, know all such books as 'herbals'.

For generations, the mighty armies of the Roman Empire spread Roman civilisation over most of the known world, and in doing so opened up those new areas for the colonial exploitation of whatever riches they possessed, whether human, animal, mineral or plant. Many new herbs from many lands became available to the Roman doctors, so many indeed that even the best-read doctors were confused.

Into that confusion, in the first century AD, there stepped an army surgeon determined to assemble in one mighty herbal all the then known information on plants and other drugs. Pedanius Dioscorides was from Asia Minor, and travelled far with the conquering armies of Nero.

A practising doctor and surgeon, he was well equipped for the task he set himself. He wrote that, as a doctor, he found it a problem that there was no definitive herbal, and that those herbals that existed not only contained gross errors, but were also incomplete. It was essential for successful treatment that a healer had sufficient and accurate information on the drugs he used. Also, that information had to be in such a form that it could readily be added to, as new plants became available for use, in the wake of the armies' expansion of all the frontiers of empire. The herbal Dioscorides envisaged had to be a solid foundation on which doctors and healers of the future could experiment and build.

His work, *Perihulas iatrakos*, is better known by its Latin name, *De Materia Medica*, or by the English title, *About Medicinal Trees*. It was instantly acclaimed and accepted. It was both the prototype herbal and the prototype pharmacopoeia, and has been issued and reissued and translated and amended ever since the good Dioscorides laid down his quill and no doubt sighed with satisfaction at having completed his task.

Although some animal and mineral substances were described and evaluated, it is the section on plants that made Dioscorides famous, and ensured that even 2,000 years later, he is revered by every herbalist who follows the western traditions of herbal healing. His knowledge was so great and his descriptive power so vivid, that every plant he wrote about could be recognised, especially since he accompanied his words with a clear little drawing. He gave details of the plant's medical uses, of how it was to be harvested, prepared and administered.

As the armies of Rome raged over the vast empire, they carefully guarded the health of their men. The army doctors and surgeons marched with the legions and carried stores of herbs from many countries, including some, such as opium and ginger, which had to be imported from distant countries. When forts and settlements were established, herb gardens were planted, and as a result plants we now regard as common or native became established in new areas. As well as the herbs themselves, the Roman doctors spread their extensive, and usually accurate, knowledge of how herbs can be used in healing both sickness and wounds. Amongst these was the invaluable garlic, for them an essential both in diet and healing.

The great Hippocrates, who lived from 468 to 377 BC, has become enshrined as the Father of Medicine. He followed one of the Greek schools of healing, that of Hygeia, and believed that both health and disease were under the influence of natural laws and that both health and disease reflected the influence of the environment. Amongst his beliefs was that we should 'let food be our medicine and medicine be our food'. Health, he believed, is a state of dynamic equilibrium among the many various factors that govern the mind and the body, and that that equilibrium can be obtained only when man lives in harmony with his environment. That belief, of course, is still, more than 2,000 years later, the bedrock upon which all holistic medicine, including herbal medicine, is based.

Although it is the one with which, in the west, we are most familiar, the basic philosophy of healing advocated by Hippocrates was by no means unique. In China, India and Egypt the great traditions of healing espoused similar views about balance – physical, mental and emotional – as being essential to health. Disease, they all held, was a disturbance of that balance, and it was the task of the healer to help the patient restore the balance. Hippocrates believed that the body had four 'humors', blood, bile, phlegm and choler, and in the healthy body these four were equally balanced. Any unbalance resulted in ill-health, and treatment must be devoted to helping restore that balance.

Four centuries after Hippocrates, the great healer Galen appeared, and it was he who laid down rigid principles and philosophies that ruled western healing for the next 1,500 years.

Galen was a native of Pergamon in Asia Minor who travelled to Alexandria to study at the great medical school there. His studies successfully completed, Galen became a surgeon to the Roman gladiators, a position which must have given him much scope and an endless supply of patients. Later he went to Rome and set up his practice there. He was a good and successful healer, so much so that he was appointed personal physician to the great Emperor Marcus Aurelius, and filled that exalted position until the Emperor, his friend and protector, died in AD 180.

By that time, Galen was rich, famous and very self-confident. He was appointed physician to the successors of Marcus Aureleus, and continued his brilliant career until, laden with honours, he died in AD 200.

Basing himself largely upon the teachings of Hippocrates, Galen established a firm philosophy of healing. However, it was a rigid philosophy, in which the healer first determined which humor was out of balance, and then prescribed the particular herb which would restore the balance. It was mechanical medicine, in which the body automatically responded to, and was healed by, the particular herb, or mixture of herbs, prescribed. It was no longer the duty of the physician to help the patient's own natural powers of recuperation: rather it was the duty of the patient to respond to the treatment. Indeed, it was not unlike the situation of medicine today, where the physician, hard pressed and short of time, treats the patient's symptoms with a drug, and ignores entirely the underlying causes of the symptom.

Galen was obviously a man capable of continuous hard work, and with a mind determined to impose a rigid order upon the art of healing. He undertook to impose that order upon the plants themselves, and in his massive *Peri kroteos Kai Danames Ton Naplon Pharmoken*, all the great many plants known to him and used in his practice were ascribed a value in changing the patient's humors. Plants were 'hot and dry', 'hot and moist in the first degree', 'cold in the fourth degree', 'cold and dry', and so on. The physician only needed to determine which humor was out of balance, and then choose from his vast armoury of plants the one which would restore that balance by adding hot or cold, dryness or moistness or any conceivable combination of them. Automatically and inevitably, the human machine was thus restored to its balance. If only healing was really as simple as that!

As the years passed, that vast Roman Empire began to disintegrate, as all empires do, and in the early years of the 5th century AD, the great soldier Alaric, leader of the Visigoths, appeared at the gates of Rome itself. In 408 and again in 409 the Goths laid siege to Rome, and then in 410 Alaric attacked and breached the defences of the city.

It was a great victory for him, and for six days the invaders were allowed to pillage the immense wealth of the city, although Alaric, a Christian himself, forbade the dishonouring of women and the destruction of religious buildings.

However, Alaric did not live long enough to impose any new order on the ruins of empire, and with his death a dark age descended. Soon, there was no-one to dispute or disagree with the teachings of Galen. Irreconcilable differences appeared between

those who followed Galen's rigid and theoretical approach to illness, and the traditional healers. To the followers of Galen, it was
only necessary to determine the heat or cold of the patient, his dryness or moistness, and then prescribe the appropriate remedy. The
traditional healers, who of course vastly outnumbered the trained
and educated followers of Galen, knew nothing and cared nothing
for the rigid classification of illness and remedy: they knew only
that the herbs they used, and which their ancestors had used,
worked well and relieved illness and helped their patients to a
restoration of health. Thus, in western medicine, began a split,
both theoretical and practical, which persists to this day, and only
in recent years are there signs that perhaps that split can be healed.

The traditional healer, and indeed also the village wise woman,
the housewife and mother and the tribal medicine man, knew that
their herbal remedies worked, but worked slowly and gently. The
professional doctor, all too often hurried and harassed, then as
now, sought quick and spectacular results. He was confident in his
knowledge, and confident that he could hurry along the processes
of nature.

It was a natural development from that mechanistic view of illness (the belief that illness was best treated by stopping whatever
symptoms there might be) to the belief that purging the body was
usually a vital step in the process of healing. Intervention in the
bodily processes themselves came to be regarded as not just desirable but as essential. Powerful drugs, animal, herbal and mineral,
were used freely and mercilessly to provoke 'evacuation' from the
sufferer's body. Evacuation of faeces, urine, saliva, blood, vomit or
perspiration, in vast quantities, was regarded as essential to
restore the balance of the humors.

Of course, this worked sometimes, and at worst, it was very
obvious that the medicines were having an effect of some kind,
and this, presumably, ensured the reputation of the doctor, and the
relief, mental at least, of the patient. Much later, this medical
determination to provoke evacuation led to the horrors of the
mercurial treatment of syphilis, where effectiveness was measured
by the number of buckets of saliva the patient evacuated daily.

In his search for effective drugs, Galen himself took one drug, theriac, and developed it into an incredible compound designed to treat virtually all illnesses and poisons. Galen did not himself invent theriac: it had already been in popular use for a hundred years. But he added to it, refined it, and constantly tinkered with it, and prescribed it so frequently that it became known as Galene. Into Galene went dozens of different herbs, many of them already themselves compounded, the flesh of snakes, various mineral compounds, opium, wine and honey. Preparing this devil's brew took 40 days, and the best of it was left to mature, like a fine whisky, for several years before it was considered ready for use.

So popular was theriac that its use and its popularity continued for around 1,000 years after the death of Galen. It continued, indeed, getting more preposterous and complicated, for all the many years that Galen's teachings and reputation lasted, and that was until Harvey showed that the blood circulated within the body, and thus destroyed the basic philosophy of Galenism. But for that 1,000 years or so, the teachings of Galen, brilliant and revolutionary though they were in his day, stultified and hindered the progress of healing in the western world. Argument or discussion about medicine and healing were effectively ended by 'But Galen said...'

Meanwhile, as the graduates of the great medical schools continued to evolve more and more complicated – and expensive – Galenical compounds, the traditional healers continued their treatments with simple herbal products, teas and beers, poultices, tinctures and whole herbs.

As the centuries passed, empires rose and fell, nations and states grew and passed away, and gradually the world developed into roughly the pattern we know today. We know it, and tend to think of it as permanent, although inevitably that pattern, too, will change. Trade routes developed, and the products of each area of the world began to be available world-wide, and trade included many herbs and other products then being used as medicines.

During long dark centuries, and also during the times of renaissance, the arts of healing, like all the other aspects of civilisation, grew and developed. However, they did not develop in harmony and co-operation. Healing split into different disciplines, and practitioners of each fought bitterly with each other to defend their territories – and, of course, their wealth. There were physicians, surgeons, barber-surgeons and apothecaries, and each sought not just to practise their skills, but to keep the others out. It was a long and indecisive battle which lasted for centuries, and the one thing that united the various professional healers was the determination, at all costs, to keep healing in the hands of the formally trained and educated, and to keep out the simple practises of the traditional healers.

And yet it was those traditional healers, with their gentle herbal preparations, and with the accumulated knowledge of a thousand generations, who were responsible for the health care and the treatment of the vast majority of the population, those who had no access to the trained doctors or who could not afford to employ them.

Throughout Western Europe, at least, the various Christian religious orders, with their great wealth and wealthy monasteries, were also centres of healing. It was the duty of the monks to care for, accommodate and heal pilgrims, and there were many of them, passing on their way to the centres of Christian grace and forgiveness. They were cared for in 'spittals' and later hospitals. From that duty, inevitably, grew the practise of treating the illnesses of all around.

Those monks, of course, had the advantage of being able to read and write. They had access to medical texts, and their monasteries had land on which herbs could be grown, and the labour and the money to do that. For generations those monasteries were responsible for the medical care of much of the population, mostly in the countryside, whilst the trained doctors and surgeons and apothecaries were concentrated in the cities and ports. Ellis Peters, in her brilliant novels about Cadfael, the monk-herbalist (or herbalist-monk), described how he carried on his task of herbal healing during one of the darkest periods of English history.

In Western Europe, as the known world grew larger, so did the choice of herbs and drugs. Many of these came from the Far East, and the Arab nations had a stranglehold on the supply of these, a stranglehold they struggled hard to preserve. All trade between the eastern world and the west had for centuries to pass through the Arab lands, and out of the vast variety of herbs available from that supply, the Arabs evolved a remarkable skill in making and compounding medicines.

This skill of the Arab apothecaries fed back to Europe. From the time of the Crusades, which were as much about trade and trade routes as they were about the holy places of Christianity, army surgeons began to learn some of the skills of the Arab apothecaries, and the Arab pharmacy had an immense effect on the prescriptions of European physicians, and also, of course, on the wealth and influence of the European apothecaries and doctors.

Many of the spices we know and use in our kitchens today were first introduced to the west from the Arab pharmacies. Nutmeg, mace, cloves and saffron are examples of our modern culinary spices first introduced and used as medicines, and indeed as effective treatments. Of course, it was not just herbs that were introduced from the east. The Arabs inherited the medical teachings of Egypt and Babylon, and, as trade across the world grew, of India and China. The European physicians benefited from this, and so did the apothecaries, whose shelves were stocked with native and imported herbs, but were also packed with strange and exotic imports. Rhinoceros and 'unicorn' horn jostled with the oil of earthworms, crab eyes, viper flesh, powdered mummy, goat urine, moss from a dead man's skull (best if it was from a hanged man), and many another unlikely thing, few of which could have had any other but a placebo effect, even when carefully compounded with a pinch of powdered pearls or the best Hymetus honey.

In spite of the Arabian apothecaries' strange exports to the vast markets of Europe, Arab medicine was for some hundreds of years the most advanced and effective available. By the 2nd century AD, the Arabs had control over the trade of the whole Mediterranean area, and a great wealth of Greek and Roman texts became available to them, many unknown to the west. They were collated and stored in Baghdad's 'House of Wisdom', and eventually translated into Arabic.

Those texts, when combined with the keen and receptive Arab mind, produced a great flowering of medical knowledge and practice, which, if only its early brilliance had lasted, would surely have had a profound effect on our philosophies of healing even to this day.

The Arabs established great teaching hospitals where medicine was taught in the wards, rather than in the lecture halls. They realised the importance of sanitation and of preventative medicine, and taught both to their students. They emphasised the importance of diet. The great healer Rhazes (865-925) wrote that 'When a cure can be obtained by diet, use no drugs, and avoid complex remedies when simple ones will suffice.' Excellent advice indeed!

Perhaps because of the great variety of herbs and other medicinal products that were available to the Arab physicians, and because of the vast profits to be made in trading and prescribing those things, Arab medicine did not for long follow the path trodden by Rhazes and his colleagues. The temptation to use complex and complicated mixtures was too strong.

Ibn Said, who in the west we know as Avicenna (980-1037), was something of a genius, and by the age of seventeen was already a successful and respected physician in Baghdad. He tended, though, to favour the teachings of Galen and not of Hippocrates, and certainly not Rhazes. Consequently, emphasis swung again, and this time decisively, to the principle of the physician controlling and curing the illness, rather than removing its cause and encouraging the body to heal itself.

Avicenna's magnum opus was a vast, million-word tome, *As-Qanum* – the Canon of Medicine. This has been described as 'the final codification of Graeco-Arabian medicine... it gave the appearance of almost mathematical accuracy... that made the medieval world regard it as an oracle from which it was impossible to dissent.'

The teachings of Avicenna and of Galen became the supreme texts for western medicine. It was as though they were carved on stone and God-given. Very understandably, those who were ill, and could afford a doctor and his expensive, complicated prescriptions, preferred the educated physician, with his armoury of exotic herbs and mysterious, evil-smelling and evil-tasting things, to the simple products of the local fields and hedgerows. Surely the expensive theriac must be more effective than anything a local wise-woman could produce, even if she had successfully treated your grandfather for the same complaint. Sadly, this is an attitude that lingers still today.

The 'evacuations' which the physicians produced in such abundance, and the blood-letting, were often spectacular, and were believed to be clear evidence of effectiveness. Fortunately, of course, many illnesses are self-limiting: like the common cold, they run their course and disappear again, till the next time, and no doubt the physicians regarded those many cases as successes for their treatments.

Even if the physicians did produce some spectacular results, if not cures, they certainly knew how to prescribe strange and expensive mixtures. One day in 1595, Queen Elizabeth's Ambassador to the Court of Henry IV of France was afflicted with severe pain in his side. The King's physicians treated him well, he later reported in a letter to his Queen. They dosed him with generous amounts of Confectio Alcarmas, 'applied a pigeon to his side and used all other means that art could devise'. The Confectio Alcarmas, a popular prescription then for those who could afford it, must have been horrendously expensive, for it was compounded of musk, amber, gold, pearls and unicorn horn. One does rather wonder where the apothecaries acquired the unicorn horn. Fortunately, the Ambassador recovered before the King's doctors really unleashed all their treatments upon him. Perhaps the pigeon did what it was meant to do, and drew the sickness out of his side. Whether the pigeon also recovered is not recorded.

It cannot be stressed too strongly, though, that throughout all the centuries of change and turmoil in the medical professions, still the mass of people had no access to professional medical help. They relied on the inherited knowledge and wisdom of the folk healer, the grandmother or the wise-woman, who knew well that meadowsweet and marshmallow soothed the digestive system and that tormentil would cure diarrhoea. They knew, even if they did not know how or why.

Moving from the wide picture of medicine and healing throughout western Europe to the situation in Britain itself, perhaps the most important factor for herbalism in those years were the changes made by royal decree during the reign of Henry VIII.

Surely no English ruler has acquired such a bad reputation over the centuries as that king. He is generally regarded as a dissolute, greedy, sex-ridden man, syphilitic, ruthless, determined to protect and prolong his Tudor dynasty at all costs, and, worst of all, the destroyer of the monasteries and the thief of their wealth.

Perhaps he was all of those things, and yet he was also, especially during the early years of his reign, an immensely popular monarch, a skilled manipulator of people and events. He had not expected to inherit the throne, being a younger son, and was still a minor when he was crowned. The throne was naturally expected to go to his elder brother Arthur. Shortly after his marriage, though, Arthur died, and in 1509 the crown passed to Henry, who promptly wed his brother's widow, Catherine of Aragon.

Henry was young – born in 1491 – and already a popular figure. Certainly he seemed to offer a profound and welcome change from the heavy-handed, heavy-taxing and generally gloomy and unpopular reign of his father, Henry VII. This new king seemed to represent youth, energy, new ideas, vigour and determination. A comparison with the election of New Labour in Britain in 1997, with a youthful and popular leader, is valid.

Henry inherited a kingdom which was itself in thrall to Rome. The Roman church was immensely powerful, and immensely rich. The monasteries in England and Scotland had by this time acquired vast land holdings and wealth which were ever increasing. The Popes had decreed, with no Biblical authority, that there was an intermediate stage between the eternal blessing of heaven for the goodly and the eternal torment of hell for the sinful. This was purgatory, another place of torment for those who did not quite qualify for either eternal bliss or eternal torment. Those souls consigned to purgatory had a second chance: they could endure their sentence there, repenting of their sins before transferring to the eternal bliss of heaven.

However, to be allowed that second chance for eternal bliss, the not-so-sinful but not altogether good, had to pay their dues to the church, and that usually entailed transferring their wealth and their land to the Church. This, and the sale of pardons for sinning, ensured that the church's wealth grew even greater, and much of this wealth was transferred to Rome by the payment of annuities each year. Henry's determination to end this haemorrhage of wealth from his kingdom to Rome was a very significant factor in the split from the Roman church, at least as great as the quarrels about divorces and the legitimacy of his marriage to his dead brother's widow.

On first ascending to the throne, Henry was a devout Catholic, so devout that the Pope awarded him the title of Defender of the Faith, and that was the Catholic faith, a title still held by the British crown to this day, and one which still creates dissension.

School children still remember Henry's complex married life, and the fate of his wives, by the rhyme:

Divorced, beheaded, died.
Divorced, beheaded, survived.

Henry had an acute and enquiring mind, and amongst his many interests was medicine and healing. It is not improbable that his own health was to some extent responsible for this interest, although other rulers, both before Henry and after, shared that interest. He had a very obstinate and troubling ulcer on his leg, and some of the ointments he himself devised were used in treating himself.

There is a manuscript which records no less than 114 royal recipes, and of these, 32 are noted as being created by the king himself. Most of them are for ointments probably meant to cure his leg ulcer, but others reflect his energetic sex life. The King's Grace Ointment was 'To cool and comforte the Member', and another was to 'Dry excoriations and comforte the Member'.

Most of the ingredients used by the king in his experiments were gentle herbs, herbs which had been used from time immemorial, and indeed are still used today in herbal practice, although generally for rather different purposes. Marshmallow, plantain and sweet violet were favourites, although exotics like powdered coral and powdered pearls also appear.

With the expropriation and then the destruction of the monasteries by Henry, a major healing resource was lost. The herbalist-monks, with their traditional herb gardens and traditional knowledge of healing, disappeared along with the carousing abbots and the drunken monks of lore. With their going also went the only source of trained help for many people – the pilgrims, the travellers, the poor and the local people.

Meanwhile, the educated, university-trained, professional healers continued their interminable battles to preserve their territories. Physicians, surgeons, barbers, apothecaries, even grocers, organised into guilds and groupings, split up, and rejoined, quarrelling, seeking Parliamentary and royal support for their profession and its profits, and united only in their detestation of the uneducated, traditional healers who remained the only source of experienced help in sickness for the mass of people.

Ultimately it was the physicians who seemed to come out on top after all the battling. By an Act of Parliament in 1543, the physicians were given control over surgeons and apothecaries, and the surgeons themselves, and their inferior colleagues, the barber surgeons, were given control over surgery in London. However, barbers were forbidden to practice surgery, even the simple blood-letting and tooth-drawing to which they had been previously confined. The only relic of the long tradition of barber-surgery is the barbers' still-used and traditional red and white striped sign, a memento of the days when they advertised their trade by flourishing the blood-soaked bandages from their shop front.

It seems to have been the surgeons who most ruthlessly pursued the unlicensed healers and invoked all the rigours of the law against them. Time and again, they acted against women who treated their neighbours, or who professed to have skill in healing, but in one case they caught an unexpected Tartar.

Most of their victims were poor and simple folk, but when they accused a brewer, Margetson, of 'giving water to cleanse men's eyes', they discovered he had powerful friends, and he fought back.

Perhaps the king himself was tired of the perpetual squabbling between the medical professions, and tired also of the constant actions against the untrained healers. After all, he was one of those himself. Parliament, provoked by the action against the brewer

Margetson, passed a new Act, ever after referred to by the medical profession as The Quacks' Charter, to protect all those unlicensed traditional healers.

The medical professions know it as The Quacks' Charter; others, still today, as The Herbalists' Charter.

In language which seems to boom and resonate, as though coming from the voice of God rather than from the pen of a Parliamentary scribe, the Act rebuked the physicians for 'minding only their own lucre and nothing the profit or ease of the diseased or patient'. They had 'sued troubled and vexed divers honest persons, as well men as women, whom God has endowed with the knowledge of the nature, kind and operation of certain herbs, roots and waters, and the using and ministering of them to such as has been pained with customable diseases, as womens' breasts being sore, a pin or web in the eye, uncomes of hands, scaldings, burnings, sore mouths, the stone, strangury, savelim and morphew, and such other like diseases, and yet the said persons have not taken anything for their pains or cunning, but have ministered the same to poor people only for neighbourhood and God's sake, and pity and charity.'

This was in contrast to the surgeons, who 'allowed many of the sick to perish for lack of help because they could not pay.' Furthermore 'the most part of the craft of surgery have small cunning, yet they will take great sums of money and do little therefore, and by reason thereof they do oftentimes impair and hurt their patients.'

This scathing attack on the skill of the surgeons and physicians, and on their morals and honesty, was followed by words that legitimised the work of the traditional healers:

> It shall be lawful to every person being the King's subjects, having knowledge and experience of the nature of herbs, roots and waters, or of the operation of same, by speculation or practice within any part of the King's dominions to practice, use and minister in and to any outward sore, uncome, wound, apostemations, outward swelling or disease, any herb or herbs, ointments, baths, poults and amplaister, according to their cunning, experience and knowledge in any of the diseases, sores, and maladies aforesaid,

and all others like to the same, or drinks for the stone or strangury, or agues, without suit, vexation, trouble, penalty or loss of
their goods.

Finally, the physicians were warned to keep their hands off the
newly legalised herbalists, whatever previous legislation might say.

Thus, in one swoop, Parliament in its wisdom, encouraged by
an enlightened monarch, provided a legal cover for the practice of
herbalism, a legal cover, which although holed here and there, is still
effective today. And all because some of the surgeons in London
attempted to harass and punish the 'divers untrained healers', and
especially one brewer, Margetson.

Although the Herbalists' Charter was directed mostly against
the surgeons, it also guaranteed herbalists the right to use some
internal medicines against some diseases. Those were specified as
'the stone, strangury and ague' – ague probably being the then
very common malaria.

This provision in fact allowed the herbalists to treat a much
greater range of illness than either a surgeon or a physician. They
could treat both internally and externally, whereas the professionals
were limited to one or the other.

The physicians of the day had no effective treatment for the
dreaded stone – small gravel-like calculi trapped in the kidney and
bladder which frequently caused excruciating pain when urinating.
The sufferers had to be passed to the surgeons for the terrifying
lithotomy operation, which only too often left the patient in a
worse state than before, and, in those days before anaesthesia,
must have been unimaginably painful.

The herbalists, though, had a considerable range of plants they
used (and still do) to treat and cure the stone. They also had many
simple preparations to treat other urinary problems, such as strangury, or pain when urinating. As to ague, or malaria, which was
very common throughout Europe in those days and was a greatly
debilitating disease, with recurrent bouts of fever, the usual herbal
treatment was with tormentil, which although slow and not very
effective, did relieve the fevers which was certainly more than the
complex and expensive concoctions of the physicians could do.

Later, as trade with the New World developed, it was found that the herb Jesuits' Bark or Peruvian Bark (from which quinine was later extracted) was a specific against malaria, and it was promptly monopolised by the physicians.

Perhaps the most significant point about the Herbalists' Charter was the recognition that traditional medicine flourished, and that there was a considerable body of men and women outside the medical professions who could and did provide a vital service, especially perhaps to the poor. Furthermore, those traditional healers had the support of influential people, right up to the monarch himself.

Inevitably, the physicians and surgeons were not totally constrained by the majesty of the law. Repeatedly the 'poor people' who used their skills to heal others were brought before the courts. In many cases they were found guilty (magistrates themselves being of the same social class as the professional doctors) and either imprisoned or enjoined to cease their activities. Sometimes, though, with the active help of powerful allies, they won their case. Even Queen Elizabeth I, herself a keen student of healing, intervened more than once to rescue some herbalist from the courts – and thereby enforced the law which her father had done so much to institute.

As time passed, another type of healer began to appear. Far from being 'poor people', these were ladies of the manor, the wives of rich landowners, sometimes aristocrats. Those women were not only the means of producing children to carry on the line – very many of whom died in infancy and so had to be replaced as quickly as possible – but also the managers of a considerable and complicated operation. The household was their responsibility, and this entailed not just the cooking, cleaning and maintenance of the establishment, but all the food production, the brewing, the distilling, the dairy, cheese making, preserving, salting, and a thousand other household requirements. Not, of course, that the lady of the manor did all those things herself, but she did supervise them, and had to have a considerable knowledge of them.

There was a great flowering of books about herbalism and the use of herbs in those days. They were at last being produced in

English, rather than the traditional Latin, of which housewives would have little knowledge, and they were devoured voraciously. Many hundreds of them have survived, mostly well used, and often with hand-written marginal notes, noting how well or poorly the various remedies acted, and also adding new recipes passed on from friends or family.

Soon another task was added to the manifold duties of the housewife, and that was to act as a medical adviser to all the people in the household and on the estate. Usually far from London, where the physicians, surgeons and apothecaries generally accumulated and continued their quarrels about who could treat what and with what, and in any case being too powerful, wealthy and influential to attack, those housewives rapidly became an invaluable medical resource for many people.

It seems safe to assume that most of the medications prescribed by those ladies of the manor would be the simple herbs found locally. Many of the books, though, also contained the complicated preparations beloved of the physicians, often handwritten, and presumably given to the housewife by a doctor. One such is described by Barbara Griggs in her wonderful book *Green Pharmacy*. It was a 'Prescription For the Head', given by the noted physician Thomas Sydenham to Lady Sedley in 1686.

This used Venice Treacle (a development of Galen's theriac), which was itself compounded from 70 ingredients and was naturally very expensive, together with wormwood, orange peel, angelica, nutmeg, all mixed together with horseradish, elecampane, scurvy grass, white horehound, centaury, chamomile and juniper berries. All of this was to be infused in five pints of sack – a wine.

It seems unlikely that Lady Sedley would prescribe and administer that atrocious and very expensive mess to the fifth undergardener who was suffering again from migraine, although possibly she would send him some feverfew leaves, which old Nanny used to use for headaches. And the under-gardener would be the better for it, although perhaps if Lord Sedley had a persistent headache, messengers would be galloped off to the apothecary shop in search of ingredients for that brew. And he would be the worse for it.

It is easy now to laugh, even sneer, at Thomas Sydenham's headache cure. In fact, Sydenham was a highly skilled and innovative doctor, so much so that he is often called The English Hippocrates. As a young man he was a brave and successful soldier in the Parliamentary Army during the Civil War, and then studied medicine at Oxford and Montpellier. His books, in Latin, were better known on the Continent than in England, although his reputation as a doctor was established in England.

He was essentially a physician, and studied his art at the bedside of the patient, rather than from books or lectures. One of his strangest, but most popular remedies was for senility, where he recommended putting the patient to bed with a vital young person! That is a treatment that surely would be popular today if only doctors could be persuaded to prescribe it. Many notable figures in history, from Solomon to Mahatma Gandhi, have used it and would perhaps vouch for its efficacy. Perhaps Sydenham's greatest contribution to medicine was his use of Jesuits' Bark in the treatment of ague, but in spite of that he held the use of herbs in contempt. It is reported that when he was told that Sir Hans Sloane was a good anatomist and botanist, he said 'Anatomy, botany – nonsense! Go to the bedside. There you can learn disease.' Later Sloane told Sydenham he planned to go to Jamaica to collect plants, and was told in return that he would be better to drown himself in St. James' Park!

Fortunately, Hans Sloane disregarded Thomas Sydenham's advice, and leaving the house the two were sharing, went to Jamaica as Physician to the Governor. In the two years he was there, he collected an herbarium of 800 native plants. Later he became one of the most successful doctors of his age, and was Physician-General to the army, and first Physician to King George II. However, he is best known, and affectionately remembered, for founding the Chelsea Physic Garden, a blessed green place in the heart of London, which still exists as a vital tool for the study of medical botany. When he died in 1753, he bequeathed his vast herbal collection and his library of books and manuscripts to the nation. They were placed in Montague House, which became the British Museum, and were the seed for probably the largest and best herbal library in the world.

One of the developments in this period was the growing practice of the apothecaries in both prescribing and administering medicines, to the great distress of the physicians. It is easy to understand why the apothecaries should extend their business that way. After all, they had long experience in compounding medicines, they were – mostly – trained, and they knew what various effects the things they sold would produce. Besides, of course, medicines from them were far cheaper than from the physicians. To the fury of the physicians, much medical practice passed to those dealers in a thousand things, some being simple dried herbs from the countryside or imported from the other side of the world, and others strange and exotic products still held to be beneficial and medically active.

One of those apothecaries, who became a healer to his neighbourhood, was Nicholas Culpeper (1616-1664). Revered to this day in herbal circles, he became an apothecary by accident, literally by a flash of lightning.

His parents had both social standing and some wealth, and Nicholas, a brilliant scholar, studied at Cambridge. However, before graduating, he fell in love and planned a runaway marriage. Sadly, his love was killed by a lightning strike on her way to the tryst at Lewes, and Nicholas was shattered. He forsook his studies at Cambridge, and became apprenticed to an apothecary in London.

After his apprenticeship and several years studying physic and astrology, he set up his own shop in Spitalfields, a semi-slum area of London, and like many other apothecaries of the day, quickly became virtually the local doctor. Unlike many others, though, he cared deeply for his poverty-stricken patients, often making no charge for his services and drugs. It was his determination to prescribe 'cheap but wholesome medicines, not sending them to the East Indies for drugs when they may fetch better out of their own gardens' – although in Spitalfields gardens must have been as scarce as doctors.

He knew well that his apothecary colleagues had become almost the only source of trained medical advice, especially for the teeming population of the growing cities. And yet those apothecaries were isolated from much medical knowledge because that knowledge was written in Latin, and few apothecaries could use them. He determined to change that by translating that knowledge into English, and in 1649 began his task with *The London Pharmacopoeia*, then the Bible of the physicians.

However, it was not a straightforward translation. He criticised, made what changes he thought necessary, and, using his own by now considerable clinical experience, advised his fellow apothecary-doctors, and any other readers of his book, on treatments. Nor did he limit his criticism of the 'proud, domineering doctors' for their indifference to the sick poor, 'those poor creatures who must forfeit their lives for lack of money'.

Perhaps worst of all, in the view of the wealthy doctors, was the fact that Nicholas Culpeper was a Puritan, and one who had fought bravely in the Parliamentary army during the Civil War, and had been badly wounded. There was a new Stuart King on the throne now, and those who had fought against, and finally beheaded, the King's royal father, were exceedingly unpopular. Most of them wisely kept their heads down, many openly repented their misguided regicidal actions, but Nicholas Culpeper refused to bow down before the torrents of reaction. Not only that, but he was exposing to public view all the closely held secrets of the medical art, so that the semi-educated apothecaries, and even, God help us, housewives and the commonest of people could read those secrets in their native English.

Just two years after the stramash caused by publication of the *Physical Directory or The London Dispensatory* – Culpeper's title for his English language version of *The London Pharmacopoeia* of the College of Physicians – he produced what was surely his greatest work, a book which was the most influential and popular herbal ever written in English. This was his *English Physician*, which he described as '...being enlarged with 369 medicines made of English herbs. A complete method and practice of Physic, wherebye a Man may preserve his Body in Health, or cure himself when sick, with such things only as grow in England, they being most fit for English bodies.'

This was an enormous and instant success, and has remained so to this day. Reprinted time after time, and still in print today, it reads rather strangely to our modern eyes. This is largely because Nicholas appeared to base his teachings on astrology. Of course, in his times there was nothing unusual in that, for astrology then formed a large part of the education of all professional healers. Nicholas wrote that 'He that would know the reason of the operation of the Herbs, must look as high as the Stars.' Nevertheless, in his recommendations for treatment of all the illnesses he described, he did not allow his astrology to interfere with the knowledge gained from his years of experience as a healer amongst the sick poor and others in London. His recommendations were terse and clear.

Writing of 'The stomach and its infirmities', he said 'Let such as have weak stomachs avoid all sweet things, as honey, sugar and the like; milk, cheese and all fat meats: let him not eat till he is hungry, nor drink before he is dry: let him avoid anger, sadness, much travel, and all fried meats: let him not vomit by any means, nor eat when he is hot.' Excellent advice indeed, and not too different from what a herbalist's patient would be told today.

Again, the reader of today is struck by the number of times Nicholas assumed that his reader would be very familiar with the herbs he described and prescribed. Of arrach (*Chaenopdium olidum*) or goosefoot, for example, he wrote that 'It is so commonly known to every housewife it were but labour lost to describe it.' He then praised the virtue of Stinking Arrach, as 'an universal medicine for the womb, and such a medicine as will easily, safely and speedily cure any disease thereof...' He went on: 'It is an herb under the dominion of Venus under the sign Scorpio: it is common almost upon every dunghill. The works of God are freely given to man, His medicines are common and cheap, and easy to be found. ('Tis the medicines of the College of Physicians that are so dear and scarce to find.)'

Again and again he wrote that he need not describe a particular herb, since it was so common and well-known. Yet today many of those very herbs, with their healing virtues so lovingly described, are either extinct or almost so. This, of course, is one of the many costs of modern agriculture, with its emphasis on herbicides and pesticides, and the determination to eliminate every plant that is not raised as a cash crop. It would be an interesting operation today to search the English countryside, Culpeper in hand, to discover how many of those virtuous and healing plants, then so common as to need no description, can still be found.

Perhaps the most important thing about Culpeper's Complete Herbal was that for the first time it brought into one place, and in English, most, if not all, of the accumulated knowledge of healing plants and their usage, and that knowledge had been slowly garnered over many hundreds of years. Later, the physician Thomas Sydenham complained that 'Nowadays every house has its old woman or practitioner, skilled in an art she has never learned, for the killing of mankind.'

Of course, even the great Culpeper had no knowledge of the vast herbal repertoire that still remained to be uncovered in much of the world. The ancient healing traditions of India and China and Siberia were unknown to him; great areas of the world remained to be 'discovered' by western nations; the vast forests and jungles of South America, with their wealth of plant life, were still virtually unknown. Indeed, they remain largely unknown to this day. However, this is not to denigrate in any way the achievement of Nicholas Culpeper. He made available to everyone who could read English, and could spare a couple of shillings, a concise and reliable summing up of herbal knowledge, and in doing that began a virtual revolution in healing.

Naturally enough, this had no effect on the work of the physicians. They continued to rely almost entirely upon the harsh, sometimes fatal, methods they had learned. Laudanum (opium) and mercury were their essential tools; bloodletting and purging their essential methods. Even the new-born were treated at once with harsh purgatives, and even the obviously dying tormented with constant bloodletting and mercurial compounds.

Rank, wealth and power were no protectors. In fact, the higher the status of the patient, the more physicians treated them, and the greater the torments they endured.

King Charles II, that Merrie Monarch, was himself a dabbler in medicine, like many others of the royal lines, earlier and later. He had a Physic Garden planted for his use, but his main interest was in studying how to extract what he thought would be the vital active element from his herbs. He boiled and distilled them, ground them, mixed them with his favourite mercury (and perhaps poisoned himself in doing so). He used antimony and vitriol, and his interest, like that of the physicians, was in the use of the newly discovered and exceedingly powerful chemical salts, not in the simple preparations of the hedgerows.

Well, he had the chance to try for himself all the powerful compounds he loved. One morning he had a seizure of some kind, perhaps epileptic. Two physicians who were present immediately drew sixteen ounces of blood from him. The rest of the royal physicians were soon on the scene and it seems that each applied his own favourite remedy. Cupping glasses and scarification drew another eight ounces of blood. An emetic (antimony) was followed by white vitriol, a purgative, followed by a purgative enema.

Not yet satisfied with the effects, they repeated the enema, with the addition of the very violent purgative Spirit of Buckthorn. The King's head was shaved and well blistered, while plasters were applied to his feet. For three days he lingered, refusing to recover (which, considering the treatment, was not surprising), or die, which is surprising. Finally he slipped away, apologising to his doctors for giving them so much trouble. One of the grieving courtiers is reputed to have commented 'It is dangerous to have two doctors: to have fifteen is fatal.'

Over a hundred years later, and on another continent, ex-President and ex-General George Washington, the Father of his Nation, awoke one night feeling decidedly ill. In true military style, he believed a bleeding would help, and a local bleeder – not a doctor – was sent for and drew about fourteen ounces of blood. During the next 24 hours, before he died, George Washington was drained of about four pints of blood, perhaps half of all the blood in his body, and this by the highly reputable physicians who flocked to his bedside. In addition, he was given two doses of mercury and a powerful purgative enema. With no apparent good effect from this, he was then given an enormous dose of calomel (chloride of mercury) and doses of antimony. Blisters were applied to his throat and the soles of his feet. Finally, poor George Washington managed to tell his doctors he wanted to be left alone to die in peace. Which he did, and in doing so provided the clearest possible warning against calling the doctors of those days if you woke in the night with a sore throat and a chill after being well soaked by a rainy day. Ironically, it was George Washington's own comrade and fellow-revolutionary, Thomas Jefferson, who wrote that the greatest service which can be rendered to any country is to add a useful plant to its culture. He could well have added that an even greater service would be to use the useful plant in healing.

And so it went on, with the physicians dispensing their 'heroic' medicine to those who could afford it; with the apothecary-doctors treating the poorer people and selling them whatever they could afford of the horrible mixtures and compounds they peddled; the housewives and ladies of the manor doctoring the household and estate workers, but now doctoring them with the new chemical emetics and purgatives found in the new medical chests which became a household essential for those wealthy enough to afford them. Those medical chests were beautiful things of brass and polished wood, with neat compartments for the calomel, jalap, essence of vitriol and the other essentials for treating the sick. There was often a book of instructions and even an enema pipe, and many apothecaries, especially in London, grew rich in providing them and their refills.

Meanwhile, the people in the countryside – at least those lucky enough to escape the good offices of the lady of the manor – continued to treat themselves and their families with the old familiar and effective herbs from the fields and the woods. In the towns and growing cities, the herb-woman was still a familiar sight, with her baskets of scurvy grass, elderberries, young nettles and whatever was in season, sold at a half-penny a handful.

Britain, and indeed most European countries, seemed to be condemned to a sort of perpetual merry-go-round on which the various branches of healing revolved, making little progress and returning time and time again to the old struggles and conflicts.

It was the New World, America, which finally broke the circle. Samuel Thomson (1769-1843) was the son of a poor, dirt-scrabble farmer in New Hampshire. Samuel was club-footed and a sickly child, and the doctoring he got was not effective. Finally, when the lad was eight years old, his father, perhaps in desperation, called in a local woman, the widow Benton, who had a reputation as a healer. Under her treatment, Samuel at last began to enjoy better health, and the precocious boy was fascinated by this and by the effect that the local plants were having on his health.

He began to study the plants, and trying the effects of them on himself and his friends. His most exciting find was lobelia (*Lobelia inflata*), which made him vomit. In later years, rich, powerful and almost idolised, the insignificant little blue-flowered lobelia remained one of his favourite herbs. As the years passed, he maintained his interest in a study of herbs, learning what he could from those of his neighbours who remembered and still used the old, simple treatments.

When his mother fell ill with measles, and the doctors came to treat her with their usual mercury, opium and vitriol, Samuel watched her misery for nine weeks until she died.

He married, and some years later watched his two-year-old daughter struggle in the throes of what the doctor called canker-rash, perhaps diphtheria. The doctor finally said he could do nothing more for the child, and that she was doomed to die in agony, struggling for every breath. Without really knowing why, he claimed, Samuel filled a bath with steaming hot water and held the convulsed little body over it. For twenty minutes, he said, and which must have seemed like hours, he continued the steaming until suddenly the child relaxed and began to breathe more easily.

This episode destroyed any last remnants of faith Samuel had in doctors and their treatments of those days. He began treating his family when they were ill, usually steaming them, and using his old friend lobelia and other herbs which he had heard about or discovered for himself.

Interestingly, the steaming treatment Samuel used is rather similar to the steaming and sweating treatments widespread amongst the First Nation Americans, or Red Indians as they were called. Before the independence of the American colonies, the few doctors, all English trained, imported with themselves all the vices and the few virtues of conventional medical practice. As a result, the immigrants died in hosts. Although several writers of the day noted the magnificent physique and great hardihood of the First Nation peoples, still they were held in such contempt by the civilised usurpers of their land that their medicines and treatments were regarded as totally useless, as the ignorant babblings of savages. Besides, those Red Indians could not cure some of the many diseases the Europeans brought with them, so obviously they had nothing to teach.

Smallpox was one such disease. It was new on the American continent, and it raged through the native people, not just decimating them but in some areas virtually eliminating them. Of course, the immigrants themselves had no cure for smallpox, but over the centuries in Europe, the people had been exposed constantly to the disease, and had developed some immunity. To them, smallpox was serious and disfiguring, but not necessarily fatal. But the death of the natives, savage and brutish as they were held to be, was held to be no great loss. Governor Winthrop, a Puritan himself, and a man of God, wrote that by the plague of smallpox, 'God has cleared our title to what we possess.'

However, the new American nation began to expand westwards, and in the great plains and mountains it was not so easy to obtain the European medicines on which they had so largely depended, and more attention was paid to the treatments of the native peoples, and to whatever of the old traditional herbal remedies the colonisers still recalled. The time was ripe for change, and Samuel Thomson was the man to lead that change, and to exploit it.

Much later, Samuel wrote that all he knew of healing was what he had learned as a child and youth from the widow Benton who had treated him when he was but a sickly lad. This was hardly true. In fact, he was widely read, and the similarities between his treatments and those of the native peoples were many – too many to be coincidence. Like the treatments of the native peoples, the treatments devised by Samuel Thomson harked back to the ancient beliefs of Hippocrates. Nature itself had great healing powers, the *vis medicatrix naturae*, and it was the task of the healer to assist this power.

Samuel and his treatments came to fame (and fortune) during

Yellow Fever epidemics which swept the eastern United States in the early 1790s. The patients he treated recovered: those of the regular physicians died. Sweating and herbs worked: calomel killed.

Samuel Thomson was not just a healer. He was also a proselytiser, and, more importantly, an early example of the Yankee gogetter of tradition and fable. It would be wrong, though, to see him as just a seeker for fame and fortune. He was a kindly man, a man who agonised with his patients, especially the children. He was determined to spread his methods as widely as possible, and in doing so came up with the idea of patenting his treatments, and then licensing as many others as possible to practice them. He had invented pyramid selling, no less.

Basing himself on the protection given by his patents, he appointed Agents in each city. Those Agents sold on the rights to 'Thomson's Improved System of Botanical Practice of Medicine'. Twenty dollars – no small sum – was the price, and for that the purchaser became a Member of the Friendly Botanical Society, and acquired the right to prepare and use for himself and his family the system of medicine Samuel Thomson had so cannily patented.

The purchaser was instructed on using the medicines and treatments, and could also buy Thomson's own *New Guide to Health or The Botanical Physician*. The purchaser of the Family Right could not only use the treatments, but could sell the scheme on to others. All the users of the Thomson Treatments had to buy their medicines from the Thomson Agents, and thus from Samuel himself, for he held the patents.

The scheme was a roaring success. It spread over the United States and Canada like a forest fire. Soon, it was estimated, half the population in some areas depended upon Samuel Thomson and his disciples for their medical treatment. Samuel himself was a genius at what we today call public relations, perhaps the first ever of a new profession. He wrote and published a regular journal and books which were reprinted again and again. At the height of Thomsonianism, Samuel claimed to have three million Practitioners, all licensed by him, and all buying their herbs from his very efficient warehouses. The insignificant little lobelia, which Samuel remembered so well from his own sickly childhood, was the most popular.

Naturally enough, the regular physicians reacted to this attack on their methods and their wealth. Organising themselves into various associations, they managed in many cities to outlaw the unlicensed and irregular practice of medicine, for which they themselves issued the licences. Heavy fines, as much as 25 dollars, were imposed on Thomsonianisn Practitioners, even for treating their own families. However, Thomsonianism was so very widespread and so popular that no mere legalities could kill it. Indeed, it was so popular and of course so successful, that several states in America actually repealed the Acts that the regular physicians had instigated, and thus restored the legality of the Thomsonian practitioners.

Samuel, who died in 1843, had lit a fire which blazed so strongly that eventually it was a major factor in ending the use of Heroic Medicine, the emetics, the purging, the calomel and antimony, which had for so long tormented so many and cured so few. However, Samuel had left no successor; he trained no-one to take over the running of that vast business, which was virtually a monopoly of herbal treatments in the US and Canada. Besides, there could have been very few people with his great charisma and public relations skills. Within a few years of Samuel's death, Thomsonianism withered away.

Meanwhile in Britain, interest in herbal medicine received a tremendous boost by the activities of John Wesley (1705-91). John Wesley was the founder of Methodism, and one of the most powerful figures in British history. The Christian sect he founded later split into several groups, but it was, and has remained, one of the most influential religious groupings in the country. More than that, though, his teachings had profound political and social effects. It has often been said, and it is true, that the Labour Party in Britain owes much more to Methodism than to Marx.

The son of well-off parents with aristocratic connections, John was ordained a priest of the Anglican order, which is not surprising, since that was, and remains the State religion. However, he and a small group of his fellows at Oxford, believed that the established Church was becoming too remote from the mass of people. He proposed that the individual and the preacher must arrange their lives according to the method laid down in the New Testament. Those who sought to do so would be Methodists.

As John Wesley's theological disputes with the Established Church grew deeper and stronger, he eventually found himself banned from the pulpit. Burning with deep zeal, he determined to go to the people. And not just to any people, but especially to the degraded masses of the cities, ports and towns.

Although the Industrial Revolution was not yet fully under way, and its worst social and human excesses still in the future, nevertheless there was already more than enough human suffering to rouse the pity and wrath of John.

Since the churches were closed to him, he was driven into the open air, and at his first Revival Meeting in Bristol he spoke to 3,000 enthusiastic people. Thus began an endless perambulation through the country. His appeal was largely to the working class, the colliers, stevedores, miners, foundrymen, weavers, spinners, fishermen, artisans and day labourers, and of course to their women folk. Every day he rode 60 or 70 miles, rose early from whatever bed he had found, and preached his sermon at 5 am, so that his listeners could hear him, and then get to their day's labour. On some occasions, in the burgeoning industrial towns of the north, he is said to have spoken to 30,000 people. It has been estimated that in his lifetime he rode 250,000 miles (including many visits to Scotland) and preached 40,000 sermons.

Not content with that, he sought to bring direct help to his listeners, and how better to do that than to help them in illness, and help, too, to maintain their health. So he wrote a book, *Primitive Physic, or an Easy and Natural method of Curing most Diseases*. He advocated using simple herbal remedies, but also a healthy diet, abstinence from alcohol, bodily cleanliness and fresh air. This rather slim volume was sold for a copper or two at his meetings, and during his lifetime went into 25 editions. Obviously, it spread very widely through the industrial working class and the agricultural labourers, and, coming from such an author, must have been very influential. It certainly prepared the way for the next great development in herbal medicine.

John Wesley grew rich from his little herbal book and from his many printed sermons and theological works, and this, as he put it, 'accidentally acquired wealth' troubled him. Before he died he distributed no less than £30,000 to charity, including the establishment and financing of a herbal dispensary in Bristol, the great sea port in which he began his mission.

There can be no doubt that the good John Wesley, with his little *Primitive Physic or An Easy and Natural Way of Curing Most Diseases*, prepared the soil and spread the seed which later grew into Coffinism.

Thomsonianism as such did not reach Britain in any strength, but a development or off-shoot of it did. This was brought by another American, the unfortunately named Dr. Albert Isiah Coffin. Born in 1790, Dr. Coffin claimed that, like Samuel Thomson, his interest in herbs had developed in his youth, and that a friendly neighbourhood doctor had helped by lending him books, which he studied avidly.

He claimed that he studied so much, and so late into the night, that his health suffered, and after a series of colds, coughs and catarrhs, finally fell ill with tuberculosis. He went down to 60 pounds in weight, he said, and the doctors expected him to die. Again, as with Samuel Thomson, fate intervened, not as the widow Benton, but as an old woman of the Seneca tribe of Indians, who came peddling baskets and brooms one day. She caught sight of the sick lad, and offered to cure him in exchange for a gallon of cider. The old woman gathered a big bundle of herbs from the woods, including, Albert later claimed, prickly ash (*Zanthaxuylum americanum*). She prepared a strong decoction of the herbs, and Albert was persuaded to drink it. He did, and almost immediately felt better, and, continuing the treatment, soon made a complete recovery.

This reprieve from death totally destroyed whatever faith he had in the conventional medicine he had studied so assiduously and which had failed him in his hour of need. He determined to travel through his country with the tribes of native Americans, learning what he could of their methods of treatment.

Albert Coffin was always rather reticent about his early years, but there was no doubt that he acquired a very considerable knowledge of herbs and their usage. Part at least of that knowledge must have come from Samuel Thomson, for Albert was at one time a Thomsonian Agent and Practitioner in New York State. Like his probable mentor Samuel, Albert was a brilliant public relations man for himself and his cause, and made no bones about publicising his successes. During a cholera epidemic in the town of Troy, he published a daily record of his successes in treating that often fatal disease, while the local newspaper could record only the deaths of those treated by the physicians of the town.

To say the least, Albert had complete faith in his own treatments, and when he, too, went down with the cholera, treated himself, as Samuel Thomson recommended, with lobelia, Composition Powder and copious amounts of cayenne pepper. He recovered, and trumpeted his recovery in his daily bulletin.

But a small town in upper New York State, and a life as a Thomsonian practitioner, was no stage for the effervescent and ambitious Albert. Samuel Thomson seemed to have the vast territory of America and Canada safely sewn up and in his pocket so far as herbal medicine was concerned. But, correctly, Albert reasoned that the Old World was ready for a herbal invasion from the New World.

Sailing for France with a considerable stock of Thomsonian products and herbs, he must have been disconcerted to discover that Europe was not the virgin territory he envisaged. The regular physicians had the profession of healing controlled very tightly indeed in France, and the law did not permit unlicensed healing. Even his precious packets of Composition Powder were confiscated by Customs Officers as being unlicensed medicines.

This in itself was rather ironic, for of all things, Composition Powder was harmless. An innocuous mixture of warming herbs, including Samuel Thomson's favourite cayenne pepper, it is still sold in a liquid form in every herbal store in Europe, and is a fine warming, sweat-inducing drink when a cold threatens, or to take the chill off a winter's night.

Making the best he could of the circumstances, Albert Coffin opened a shop to sell his remaining stock of herbs (that, at least, was still legal), and proceeded to learn what he could of local herbalism from the local people. However, things did not go well with him, although he did find time to marry, and finally a burglary robbed him of most of his money, so he decided to leave unfriendly France and seek fame and fortune elsewhere.

And where better to go than what he described as 'dark, physic-laden, pill-swallowing England'?

He was right, of course. It was in England that those dark satanic mills of the Industrial Revolution first began to grind. Great new factories were being established in northern England and southern Scotland, and the insatiable demand for labour was sucking in many thousands of people from the countryside. They lived in incredible squalor, crowded in buildings hastily and poorly erected for them, and were at one stroke removed from the fields and hedgerows where grew the medicines they and their ancestors had known and trusted. Not only did those Children of the Dead End welcome Albert Coffin and his herbal treatments, but they welcomed him with very open arms.

Or least they did when Albert Coffin's enormous skill as a self-publicist, as well as a herbalist, became evident. He was an entertaining and brilliant lecturer. Soon his lectures in the squalid towns of the industrial north were attracting thousands of listeners.

He was wise enough to not settle at first in London, where the medical professions, still squabbling amongst themselves, were well entrenched and united only in their detestation of unlicensed practitioners. Besides, there were many traditional and untrained herbalists already working there, and even the poorest of the poor could still treat themselves with a handful of herbs from the herb-woman on the street corner. By and large, the medical professions shunned the vast new towns of the industrial north – there was little prestige to be gained there, and little money to be accumulated.

Albert Coffin made no bones about it: he modelled Coffinism on the pattern established in America by Samuel Thomson. He set up his main herb warehouse in London, for London then was England's major port, well-equipped and experienced in handling bulk herbs. Soon he was importing great quantities of herbs, some of them novel in England, especially those from America, but also other more familiar ones from Europe and Asia.

And where did he find the market for his herbs? Simply by following Samuel Thomson's example, that is by appointing Agents and establishing 'Friendly Botanico-Medical Societies' in virtually every one of the pullulating industrial towns of northern England. The members of those organisations bought his herbs, studied his writings – which were many – and practised herbalism as he taught it.

He was, though, not just a brilliant exponent of public relations, and an astute business man: he was also a brilliant herbalist and healer. Moreover, he was a skilled teacher, and a large number of his Agents and Practitioners themselves became highly skilled and very successful herbal healers.

No small part of Albert's success was due to his appeal to the wives and mothers. Himself a teetotaller, at every one of his well-attended meetings he preached the virtues of total abstinence from alcohol, and since drunkenness was prevalent, not surprisingly, in the unutterable squalor of those industrial towns, abstinence appealed to wives and mothers. Many women themselves became Coffinite Practitioners.

His fortnightly *Journal* had a circulation of 10,000, and his Herbal Guide was reprinted twenty times. As the forest fire of Thomsonianism had spread through North America, so did Coffinism spread throughout England, and soon through the industrial belt of southern Scotland.

Albert Coffin was no doubt a very astute business man, as was his mentor Samuel Thomson, and soon he was living in a fashionable and expensive part of London. However, he was also an untiring crusader for the better health of all. His *Journal* constantly berated the physicians for their continuing use of the harsh chemical drugs they employed, and campaigned against medical interference with natural processes, such as the common lancing of babies' gums to 'assist teething'. He advocated a simple, wholesome diet, and his anger was aroused time and time again by the then common adulteration of foodstuffs. I tremble to think what he would have had to say about the fast foods of today!

Almost every issue of his *Journal* described some case where a poor patient had been subjected to the full armoury of conventional treatment, the mercury, opium and antimony, and was hovering near death, only to be saved by the administrations of a Coffinite Practitioner with the simple herbs and simple living that he taught and used. Albert was not only a superb business man and a public relations expert (and soon a very rich one), but was also himself a highly skilled herbalist who had a large practice. Night after night, after a full day in his clinics, he sat at his desk writing his *Journal* and other publications, spreading the word in which he believed so strongly. He may well have been wealthy, but he was also extraordinarily hard working.

Inevitably, of course, the medical professions began to pursue him, even though a good number of medical men were themselves converts to his cause. Indeed, Thomas Harle, a very experienced surgeon, became Albert's right-hand man after attending one of his vast public meetings in Manchester. He had gone there to jeer, but became a very enthusiastic convert.

Just a few years earlier, Adam Smith, in his seminal *The Wealth of Nations*, wrote that: 'People of the same trade seldom meet together, even for merriment and diversion, but the conversation ends in a conspiracy against the public, or in some contrivance to raise prices.' It is not known whether or not Adam Smith had the medical profession in mind, but there is no doubt that as soon as the medical professions became organised, they began seeking to eliminate all opposition, and especially the opposition posed by the herbalists.

Attacks on Coffinism were mounted at first through the law, but they found that the Quacks Charter of Henry VIII still gave the herbalists considerable clout. However, apothecaries still required a licence from Apothecaries Hall, and this the Coffinites did not have, and certainly would not be given. So most of the legal attacks on Coffinites and Coffinism were mounted by apothecaries. But to their considerable discomfiture, the orthodox medical professions found that often enough magistrates, juries and even judges were themselves enthusiastic about Coffinite treatments, and refused to convict.

None of this could have happened if Albert's treatments and herbs had not been effective and greatly popular. But they were effective, and repeatedly patients and even some doctors testified that they were, and that conventional treatment was not.

Today, much of what he advocated, used and taught seems self-evident. There really was no need to force-feed the new-born with castor oil or calomel. Rye bread was, and is, a better medicine than a chemical purge or an enema for what was regarded as the almost universal English constipation, and was in fact a truly iatrogenic problem, one, that is, caused by laxatives and purgatives. Children should be encouraged to run and play and to be in fresh air, although there was little enough of that in an industrial city slum.

It was always the treatment of babies and children that most aroused Albert's ire, and caused him most frustration. Babies, and there were a great many of them in those industrial slums, were usually weaned as soon as possible, and struggled to grow on what was a very unsuitable and inadequate diet. The mothers, of course, needed to return as soon as possible to the mills and looms where they worked. The few shillings they earned were essential to clothe and feed the family. As soon as it was weaned, the child was usually packed into some slum room, to be cared for by a hard-pressed woman, herself often a washer woman or a seamstress, augmenting her paltry income with a few coppers each week by caring for her neighbours' babies. It was tempting, and too easy, to keep the children quiet and usually asleep, by dosing them with some soothing syrup from the local apothecary or the corner shop.

Those soothing syrups, though, were always opium in one form or another, and certainly a few spoonfuls of Godfrey's Cordial and then a dummy smeared with some other soothing syrup would quieten the most fractious or hungry baby.

Many of those children grew up, if they survived at all, as sickly opium addicts, frequently stunted and with the typical yellowish skin of the addict and the sufferer from chronic constipation. It was indeed ironic and tragic that the herbalists, with their regime of healthy diet and living, and their gentle herbal treatments, were so often harried through the courts, while the doctors, with their pernicious chemical products, were almost venerated, and the apothecaries, selling their bottles of laudanum, were respected members of society, and the old women with their little corner shops, peddling pennyworths of opium extract to weary and anxious mothers, were regarded as useful conveniences.

In his continuing, but ultimately hopeless, battle against the medically approved onslaught on the health of children, Albert Coffin was faced by greater odds than even he imagined, and greater than he could ever overcome. Not only was he facing the ranks of the medical professions and the apothecaries, he was also trying to overcome the very system which produced the evils he fought. Mothers had to work, or families starved. There was no alternative to handing infants over to baby-minders. The growth of industry demanded much cheap labour. Women and children largely supplied this, working their looms and mills for long hours every day. To change the effects, he would have had to change the very system itself, and that he could not do.

Perhaps the greatest vindication of the Coffinite treatments came during the cholera epidemics which swept through the industrial towns of England in the mid-19th century. Spread by contaminated food and water, cholera was indeed terrifying in the speed with which it killed. A man could be healthy in the morning and dead at night, after suffering agonising stomach cramps and a diarrhoea so powerful that eventually only water and flakes of intestine lining could be voided. Over 55,000 people died of it in the epidemic of 1848-49, and the physicians were helpless. We know now that it is a disease of dehydration, in which the body voids all its water and its various salts, until the heart loses its stimulation and fails. It is not difficult to treat, given adequate supplies of clean water and alkaline salts with potassium.

Certainly the physicians were helpless. Their prescriptions of calomel and opium were useless, and their bleeding and purging (!) worse than useless. Those patients lucky enough to be treated by Coffinites were given copious water to drink, and various soothing herbal drinks. Enemas of various herbs were used, chiefly those with an astringent effect. If necessary, there was a lobelia emetic, and soothing drinks of arrowroot and slippery elm. Simple enough, and cheap enough, and they worked.

Later, a Commission set up by the College of Physicians investigated the epidemic, and sought to discover which of their treatments were most successful. There were none. Only the Coffinites and the growing number of homeopathic doctors, with their camphor treatment for cholera, had any record of success in treating cholera, but the Commission Report failed to mention this.

Sadly, just like his mentor Samuel Thomson, Albert Coffin refused to move with the times. It seems that even he, who should have known better, regarded his own tome *The Botanic Guide to Health*, as the final word on herbal treatments, in spite of the leaping and bounding of new knowledge in physiology, anatomy, and, most important, pharmacognosy and pharmacology, the sciences of the description of plants and of the action of medicinal substances. Greater knowledge should obviously have initiated changes in the herbs used and in how both the traditional and newly available ones should be used. Albert Coffin was blind to all of this.

Precisely the same problems had afflicted the Thomsonians in America. Like Albert Coffin, Samuel Thomson was convinced that his treatments were the last possible word and that the sciences in fact were a danger, since they made a mystery out of what was startlingly clear – that herbs cured illness. To dilute that certainty with a scientific understanding of how they cured would be to take away from the people themselves the accumulated knowledge of centuries. It was patients that should be studied, not books or theories.

In fact, the anti-intellectual beliefs of both Thomson and Coffin were the last flickering of an ancient and most noble tradition, going back thousands of years to prehistory, when the shamans and healers observed their patients very closely, and treated them according to what they saw. A fever responded to this herb and a cough to that. It was certainly not necessary to know how or why. It had always worked before, and would work again, and it was a method that could be used by anyone, trained or not, educated or not.

Empires, states and dynasties rise and then fall. Every ageing emperor – or bull – is challenged eventually by a youngster. Every Caesar has his Brutus. In the case of Samuel Thomson, the role of Brutus was played by Wooster Beach, and Albert Coffin was felled by John Skelton.

Wooster Beach, another American, was a man of great integrity, with a high moral code, at least at first. He was filled with horror at the methods and consequences of Heroic Medicine, and felt that somewhere there must be an alternative, a gentler and a more effective method of treatment. He learned of one old German doctor, Jacob Tidd, practising in New Jersey, who had gained a great local reputation by successfully treating his patients with no more than gentle local herbs.

Eventually, after he had unsuccessfully applied several times, Dr. Tidd (who was a qualified physician) agreed to take on Wooster Beach as a student-apprentice. They worked together for some years, and Wooster absorbed every scrap of knowledge he could from the doctor's lifetime experience of treating illness with herbs.

Later, Wooster himself became a qualified physician, reasoning that, if he was to reform and end the horrors of Heroic Medicine, he had better have a formal qualification allowing him to practise, and thus escape the continuing legalistic harassment suffered by unqualified practitioners.

Far from holding the anti-intellectual prejudices of Samuel Thomson and his followers, and far indeed from believing that Samuel had enunciated the last words on herbal medicine, Wooster had a receptive outlook and was willing to use and adapt newly acquired knowledge of scientific research to the practice of herbal healing. He reasoned that Thomsonianism had itself become the greatest barrier to herbalism, and that although Samuel Thomson was a great, almost instinctive, healer, the mass of Thomsonian practitioners were not, and were simply mechanically following The Word as handed down by Samuel.

Besides, Thomsonianism had become almost a monopolist supplier of herbs, and this greatly limited the development of herbalism. Furthermore, although they certainly cured most of the patients, the Thomsonian Treatments, with their emetics, their sweating and hot drinks, could be exceedingly unpleasant to follow for a suffering and debilitated patient. Certainly they were effective, but they could be almost as unpleasant to endure as the chemical compounds of the physicians, which generally did not work. As Plutarch had remarked two thousand years earlier, 'I see the cure is not worth the pain.' Wooster contrasted those treatments with the gentle herbal infusions and decoctions and poultices he had studied with Dr. Tidd, which were equally effective, and of course were much cheaper. It was that road he determined to follow. And, of course, that meant that Wooster had to fight on two fronts, that of the regular physicians and also against the Thomsonians, with their reliance, as he saw it on the 'ignorance, prejudices and dogmas of a single individual'.

It was not easy, and soon Wooster found himself under attack by his fellow physicians. He must have possessed a considerable fortune, and he published many pamphlets and periodicals, all advocating his new, gentler medicine. And so, the physicians reasoned, he must be another of those medical non-conformists, a Botanical Practitioner, and as such must be crushed.

He defended himself vigorously from the attacks, and denied that he was just a herbalist. He was, he said, an eclectic, one who selected and used the best of various ideas and methods. He would call his new system of medicine Eclecticism.

Slowly he gathered disciples from the medical profession, and was able to open a hospital in New York. Rather grandiloquently, he named it the United States Infirmary, where there would be 'introduced a new and better system of medical and surgical practice ...for the treatment of disease by a new and improved method'. The medicines 'would be derived chiefly from the vegetable kingdom', and the poor would be treated free. He did not, it may be noted, exclude altogether the use of chemical medicines.

A little later, Wooster enlarged his hospital to include a teaching facility which he named, again grandiloquently, the Reformed Medical College of the City of New York.

However, the anti-Beach forces were powerful, and the State refused to recognise the College. Wooster could not grant degrees, and the most his graduates could achieve was membership in the Reformed Medical Society of the United States, and not the accepted medical degree he sought. The New York medical professionals, united only in their detestation of herbal medicine and in their determination to maintain their medical monopoly, were powerful enough to do that. Wooster sought a qualification that would be accepted and recognised, not merely a piece of parchment really no different from that flaunted by the Thomsonian Practitioners. So, like so many others, he decided to up-stakes and migrate westwards to Ohio, his native State. There, in a more pioneering environment, the medical professions were fewer, and not so well entrenched and powerful.

He found a small college there, very run down, but which still had the power to grant degrees. He bought Worthington College, and converted it into a medical school and herbal treatment centre, practising what he of course called Eclecticism. It was a great success, and soon qualified Eclectic Practitioners, with a parchment issued by a regular and accepted College, were increasingly common throughout the United States.

Whilst all this was happening, poor old Samuel Thomson was under attack from all directions. His movement was splintering and disintegrating, and he was old and tired. He died in October 1843, and with his death America lost a great healer and a great revolutionary, but one who, like so many revolutionaries, refused to move onwards and accept that times change and knowledge increases, and that what was once progressive becomes regressive and reactionary.

Much the same process was taking place in England, and there the changes were led by John Skelton, who was born in 1806 in Devon, the son of reasonably well-off parents. Like both Samuel Thomson and Albert Coffin, John Skelton learned about herbs and their healing powers from an old woman, a healer and a midwife. She was his grandmother, and regularly took the child with her when she went gathering the herbs she used. She talked to him, taught him where the herbs grew, when they should be gathered, and how she used them in treating the sick of the village. They were lessons he was never to forget, and in later life he referred to his grandmother time and time again as his greatest inspiration and teacher.

After a sound education, John never contemplated any other profession than that of being a medical herbalist. He set up a practice and was soon a successful herbalist, with a good reputation. When Albert Coffin's fame began to spread, John was immediately interested, and when the two met, he was persuaded to join the

Coffinites. Perhaps already staggering under his colossal work-load, Albert was seeking someone to carry some of his burdens, and chose John Skelton, with his already considerable personal reputation, to be that deputy.

John was despatched to the industrial north of England, and was an immediate success, both as a healer and as a guardian of Coffinism. There could surely have been no place more in need of medical help. The Industrial Revolution was well underway, and those northern English towns its very epicentre. The new mills and factories demanded labour, and people flocked to them. The resultant towns were veritable hell-holes. In Lancashire alone, the population increased ten-fold in eighty years, and dwellings (they could not be called homes or houses) were thrown up to accommodate them. They were crowded together as close as possible, with no facilities for ventilation, drainage or water, except the occasional hand pump from a polluted well. Whole extended families existed in one room bare of all furnishings except a heap of rags for a bed. Chickens and pigs shared the accommodation, and rooted through the ordure. And all was cloaked in a constant miasma of coal smoke and factory fumes. Altogether, it was a hell on earth. The Clouded Hills of the song were a reality, and the clouds covered a depth of human misery and degradation never seen before or since. The people urgently needed medical help, but no trained doctor would dream of setting up practice there. The Coffinites did, and should be honoured and remembered for doing so.

Already Albert was aware that the younger men of his movement, themselves successful healers, had begun to question his leadership and his immutable insistence that his methods and his treatments were the last possible development, and that Coffinism was the ultimate form of healing. Some of his trusted lieutenants were already leaving him. After some time, John Skelton followed them, and in 1850 went to Edinburgh and established his own successful practice and dispensary. However, Albert Coffin persuaded him to return to the fold, and sent him to propagate the movement in Wales.

Very shortly it became clear to John that Albert really only wanted him out of the way, and in a place where he posed no threat to Albert's own leadership – almost the dictatorship – of the movement.

So John Skelton returned to the north of England, but this time in direct competition with Albert and his organisation. In a very short time, he had established not only a highly successful herbal practice, but also a considerable business in importing and processing herbs. And, like Samuel Thomson and Albert Coffin himself, he recruited others to act as Agents, practising herbalism and buying their herbs from him.

Perhaps worst of all, from Albert's viewpoint, was the writing and publishing of a monthly magazine, which was itself an innovation for it was meant to be bound together as *Dr. Skelton's Botanic Record and Family Herbal*. John had invented the still popular part-work.

Meanwhile, Dr. Wooster Beach was seeking new fields to conquer, virgin territory to exploit. Even the vast, still empty spaces of the United States and Canada were not enough for him. Where better than Europe? He was a new prophet, with his Eclectic Medicine, and, most important, with the power to grant his followers and students the much-desired degree of Medical Doctor from his Reformed Medical College in distant Ohio.

Wooster was the last in that remarkable series of herbal practitioners to come from the West back to the Old World. He followed the path first trodden by Samuel Thomson and Albert Coffin. The stage was set, and what was almost a Greek Tragedy began.

First touring Europe and successfully preaching his Eclectic Medicine there (and being highly rewarded for his success as a healer), he settled in England. He brought with him a new ruthlessness and determination. Unlike John Skelton and the other critics of Coffinism, who still respected the achievements of Albert Coffin and were still influenced by Albert's great charisma, Wooster Beach went straight for the jugular of the old man.

In his copious writings he accused Coffin and the Coffinites of bringing the cause of medical reform into disrepute, of being illiterate quacks, of being hidebound to the past, of ignoring all scientific research and in general of being not only outdated, but a positive hindrance to progress.

John Skelton had met and been impressed by Wooster when he first arrived in London, and accepted the idea that if herbalism was to flourish, it must accept and use the results of scientific research. Ideally, herbalism should strive for acceptance by the medical professions, as well as by the sick and ailing. It seemed that in the United States that was being achieved to some extent as Eclecticism gathered converts and exponents from the ranks of conventional medicine. Besides, surely a proper formal education at a properly established Medical School, and the gaining of an acceptable qualification, was the way to go. Eclecticism, John grew to believe, was the way of the future: Coffinism, like Thomsonianism before it, was the way of the past.

It fell to John Skelton to deliver the fatal blow, and ironically, the forum in which that gentle Brutus struck was in a public meeting in Bradford, the heartland of Coffinism. Albert was to address one of his public meetings there. However, when Albert saw one of the handbills advertising the meeting, he found that John's name also appeared, and was printed as prominently as his own. This was hardly surprising, for John Skelton was immensely popular there, both as a practitioner and as the man who had built up the Bradford Botanical Society in the town. Infuriated, Albert cancelled the meeting, and proceeded virtually to excommunicate John Skelton and others from his movement. Indeed, he attempted to form an entirely new Medico-Botanical Society in the town, and planned to publicise it with a public meeting.

When that meeting took place, it was both a fiasco and a tragedy. It was packed with John Skelton's supporters, and Albert simply could not handle it. He had lost the skills which had vitalised so many in the past, and which had indeed revitalised the whole herbal movement throughout the country.

He hesitated, stammered, sought the sympathy, even the pity, of his audience. They listened, but they finally rejected him. So leadership of the Botanic movement in Britain passed to the excellent John Skelton, who was by this time calling himself an Eclectic.

Not only an excellent healer himself, he was also an excellent teacher and a highly efficient organiser, with a clear understanding of the direction in which herbal medicine had to go. For one thing, it had to recognise and absorb and utilise new scientific under-standing of the human body, its workings and its ailments. It had to accept that there were other successful treatments – homeopathy, for instance. Never again must it allow itself to be subject to a monopoly either of teachings or of herbal supplies. Never again must it be bound by a rigid orthodoxy, and subject to the teachings or the whims of one person, however brilliant that person might be. Never again must herbalism be solely a vehicle for the enrichment of an individual.

With one blow, John Skelton finally killed off Coffinism in Britain, and by the force of his personality and his vision, laid down principles which governed the practice of herbalism for a hundred years.

Of course, Coffinism in Britain, like Thomsonianism in America, did not die instantly. It lingered, but without the great impetus provided by Albert Coffin, its fate was ordained.

The early years of the 19th century were an exciting period for the chemists and pharmacists. Many, if not yet most, physicians had begun to realise that there was indeed something basically wrong with the Heroic Medicine they had been educated and trained to follow. All too often, the results were obviously worse than the illness itself, and the cures were few. Not that the trained physicians of the day gave up their Heroic Medicine easily. Simply to abandon it would be to admit that they themselves had been totally wrong, and their teachers and predecessors for hundreds of years had been wrong. They needed something that could be pre-sented as a scientific reason for abandoning so much that they had used so profitably and for so long. After all, science was the new religion, and so a scientific explanation was required. Convoluted and verbose arguments in the exalted language of pseudo-science were put forward. The very nature of illness had undergone a sea-change, it was said. Fevers, which were once inflammatory in nature and so required blood-letting, had changed their character. They had changed to being of a typhoid character and so blood-letting could be fatal. 'There are waves of time through which dis-ease prevails in succession. We are at present living amid one of its adynamic phases.'

Justifying themselves with such preposterous mumbo-jumbo, the physicians put aside their lancets for bleeding, their cupping glasses and scarifiers, and began clearing their shelves of the calomel and vitriol. They began looking again at the gentler methods they had previously rejected.

The search was on for new, gentler medication, and the obvious place to seek was in the vegetable kingdom. After all, even the most purblind and hidebound physician had to recognise that the wide-spread herbal treatments did work – they saw that for themselves every day.

It was natural, then, that the chemists were encouraged to research herbs. However, it was argued that there must be some single vital principle in the herbs, and it was that single principle that did the healing. The rest of the plant was just dross. The search was on for that single herbal constituent. Besides, those crude herbs could never be prescribed with the precision the physicians were beginning to seek. They varied from supplier to supplier, and from spring to winter – a fact that the herbalists themselves recognised and allowed for. What was more, and most important, there was no way that crude herbs could be patented and monopolised. But if the vital principle could be extracted, then that could be patented and the patent exploited to the great profit of the supplier. That is a fact that continues to bedevil the pharmaceutical industry even today, and only now are they beginning to find a solution to it. If the plant can be genetically modified in some way, then that genetically modified plant can be patented, and so exploited, to the great benefit and profit of the industry.

Their reasoning was quite correct, of course, except for one vital fact. A herb does not contain just one active constituent together with a mass of dross. Each plant is an exceedingly complex and self-contained chemical factory, with many constituents, all acting and interacting with each other. To isolate one constituent is to remove all the modifying and balancing effects of those other parts of the plant. To do so is also to ignore the phenomenon of synergism, by which the sum of the plant compounds is greater than their individual separate effects, a phenomenon which is of course by no means confined to the plant world, but is also used by every chemist who mixes two drugs together to achieve an effect greater than either would give separately.

The most commonly cited example of this is the familiar dandelion, a diuretic herb used for countless generations by herbal healers. The diuretic principle of the dandelion can be isolated and removed, purified and eventually even synthesised as a powerful diuretic. But a patient treated with that extracted or synthesised diuretic is soon in further trouble from a lack of potassium and other vital salts. So the patient must be supplied with those vital salts, again to the financial benefit of the manufacturers. However, the whole dandelion plant is rich in those very salts. A patient treated with the whole herb, or an extract from the whole herb, has no need for those chemical additives. And what is true of the simple dandelion is true of virtually the whole vegetable kingdom.

All of this in no way denies that there have been some invaluable drugs extracted from plants. Opium is a case in point. Opium has been used for treatment and recreation for countless generations. Wars were fought to impose it on unwilling peoples; whole national economies have been based on it; whole nations, including our own, have been so addicted to it that the very framework and future of society was threatened. In the 18th and 19th centuries, countless thousands of babies were born already addicted through their mother's blood, and if they survived, maintained the addiction through the popular and cheap medicines they were given.

The opium poppy was one of the first herbs the chemists turned to. Research into opium continues to this day, and more than 40 different active ingredients have been isolated. The first was morphine, perhaps the most powerful, effective and addictive of all painkillers. Morphine, or morphia, was named after Morpheus, in Greek mythology the god of sleep and dreams, and when morphine was itself subjected to the alchemical magic of the chemists, other subdivisions were found. The first was named narcotine, from the Greek *norke*, or numbness, and although it was also a very powerful painkiller and even anaesthetic, it seemed to offer no great advantages over morphia, and it is rarely produced today.

The search continued, and soon heroin was isolated from the

crude opium. Now there was a great jackpot. It was so powerful that it was named the 'hero'. As a narcotic it was unsurpassed, and only had one serious drawback: it was very highly addictive, so much so that even the Heroic Physicians, those who still remained, hesitated about using it, and up to today it is used medically only in extremis, when a patient is undeniably edging towards death, and is in such pain that even morphine becomes ineffective.

But it had been isolated from its parent opium, and only too soon the results became evident. Heroin addiction became widespread, with the results we see today, when that addiction, and the illegal heroin trade, and the fight against that trade, menaces whole nations, and even challenges the national budget in some cases.

Even at that, the riches of the opium poppy were not exhausted. The popular codeine, which we buy in various forms from the local pharmacy, is a more gentle painkiller than the morphine from which it is prepared. Papaverine is a useful antispasmodic, and other constituents are still being investigated. All of that from the simple, rather beautiful, poppy.

Opium itself had certainly been grossly misused, not so much by those addicted to it as by the rich companies which forced it, quite legally, onto often unwilling people. Enormous fortunes were made from it, and in particular the traders in Hong Kong gathered wealth beyond computation from it, forcing its free use onto the Chinese. The government of China, weak and disunited, was unable to withstand the might of the traders, backed up when necessary by the military might of the Western armies. It was argued that the whole economy of India, that jewel in the crown of the British Empire, depended on opium grown for export to China – and, of course, for consumption in India and for export to the pharmaceutical factories of England.

Generally, the addicts were quiet and docile, and the careful spreading of the addiction helped to produce a quiet and docile workforce. This was true especially in colonial India, China and the United States. Aldous Huxley, in his 1932 novel *Brave New World*, caught the essence of that when he wrote of how, in some future time, the workers after each day of intensive labour for the profit of their rulers, were each, if they deserved it, given a dose of *soma*, which produced a very desirable dream-like state in which misery and injustice were forgotten. Just like opium, in fact.

On the other hand, opium has been instrumental in producing many great works of art and literature. No heroin addict has produced a vision of Xanadu with its stately pleasure dome and maidens with dulcimers, nor are they likely to. But opium has.

Having succeeded so brilliantly in dissecting opium, the chemists used the same skills and methods on other herbs, which we still call simples, but which have proved to be anything but simple. The chemists, those modern-day alchemists, showed the incredible complexity of familiar plants, which herbalists had used for their healing properties for thousands of years.

Aspirin came from the willow and from meadowsweet, but there was a downside to that, just as there was from the products of opium. Aspirin is an acid, and can cause stomach irritation and even haemorrhage. The simple plants do not, and yet they still give relief from pain and fever.

Quinine was extracted from Peruvian Bark, or Jesuit's Bark, and ended the fever and pains of malaria in Europe and much of Asia and Africa.

And so it went on, with dozens of plants being investigated and dozens of new alkaloids, as they were called, being extracted from them. The next stage was to discover the precise chemical makeup of those alkaloids, and then to duplicate it in the laboratory, and then in the factory. Soon it seemed that the factory would replace the physic garden as the source of all medicines. And those chemical medicines would be pure and concentrated. Most of all, they could be patented, and would surely be immensely profitable. And so it has proved to be.

Physicians, many of them sickened by the excesses and failures of Heroic Medicine, turned instead to the neat packets of tablets and liquids that soon poured in torrents out of the factories of the new pharmaceutical industries. Today, that great flood of medication still pours out of the factories, and the physician, probably tired and harassed and with a full waiting room, almost automatically scribbles a prescription for one of them, attempting to treat the symptom which the patient believes is his illness. Meanwhile, the apothecary became the pharmacist, who no longer dispenses, but merely trades in pre-packed packets of tablets.

Armed with their new chemical weapons, the physicians in Britain and America began to seek new powers of control over the practise of medicine and the healing arts. In 1854, a Medical Reform Bill was discussed in the British Parliament, with the object of making illegal the practise of medicine except by a regis- tered practitioner, and since the only registered practitioners were the products of the medical schools, the Bill would at one stroke destroy the practise of herbalism, and also the increasingly wide- spread practise of homeopathy.

For the first time, but not the last, the sponsors of the Bill were shocked by the response. Petitions poured into Parliament protest- ing at this attempted monopolisation of medicine. The Members of Parliament were deluged with letters of protest from simple folk as well as from the great and powerful. Most important, perhaps, many Members of Parliament were themselves users of other treat- ments than those offered by the physicians. For the first time, but again not the last, the Bill was defeated.

It was just as well that it was. At the time, there were just over 5,000 certificated members of the medical professions, and that included surgeons and apothecaries. It was calculated that there were more than 6,000 unlicensed practitioners, and also a vast and uncountable number of traditional healers, not organised in any way, but using the herbal treatments learned from the grand- mothers and Wise Women. And of course there were still the Ladies of the Manor, the wives of estate owners and the wives of ministers, who ministered to the body while the husband attended to the souls and sins of his congregation. If all those unlicensed practitioners had been compelled by law to cease their activities, a large part of the population and large swathes of the country would have had no medical help at all, for the doctors practised in London and other cities where the money and the living was easy: there were few in the industrial towns, and virtually none, for example, in the Highlands of Scotland.

One good thing did come out of that aborted Parliamentary Bill. The herbalists realised at last that they must combine into some organisation which could speak for them all and which could perhaps, in the future, engage in education, and training, and even registration in the profession.

The majority of petitions to Parliament about the proposed Bill, and the mass of letters of protest, came from the Friendly Medico-Botanic Sick and Burial Society. That organisation was an interesting early form of medical insurance, based on the principles of co-operation then becoming so popular and later so powerful. The ideas of Robert Owen and other pioneers of co-operation were applied in the Society, wherein the members, for a few coppers each week, received medical services and medicine from appointed herbalists, and also received help with the costs of burial, thus avoiding the shameful fate of being buried by the Parish as a pauper in Potter's Field. Based in the industrial towns of northern England and southern Scotland, the Society had many members, with John Skelton as one of the leaders and herbal practitioners. It was John Skelton who encouraged the Society members to protest in their thousands, and to provide a very early example of what would today be described as stake-holder power.

Herbalists have always been free spirits, and it has never been easy to persuade them to organise, even in their own defence and best interests. Furthermore, there has always been a tendency for herbal organisations to split into sects, and such schisms have been many. At the time of that first Parliamentary Bill there was the National Medical Reform League, based in London, and spreading the word that 'the treatment of disease by simple herbs, roots and barks... has proved far more safe and effective than the mineral and depletive practice'. That London-based body developed into the British Medical Reform Association, with a well-known herbalist, Mr. Ford of Derby, as its President. Albert Coffin played no part in this new Association, and very soon death claimed him, a sad and embittered old man, but one who should certainly not be forgotten. His contribution to the art of herbal healing was enormous, and herbalism has never again achieved the great popularity that it had in the industrial north under the guidance of that remarkable man. The herbalism he taught and practised was very different from that of the Thomsonians, with their arduous

Treatments and emetics and large hot drinks of usually foul-tasting mixtures. Albert Coffin reverted to the gentler, simple healing he had experienced as a child, and the profession of herbalism was the better for it.

It was the British Medical Reform Association which became the organised voice of herbalism in Britain, and was the direct ancestor of today's National Institute of Medical Herbalists.

In the United States, it was the Eclectics who made most progress, but who finally succumbed to the same faults as the Thomsonians. They became perhaps too ambitious, and attempted to monopolise Botanic healing and also to monopolise the herbal medications. At their height, the Thomsonians had been powerful enough to succeed in persuading many American states to repeal all the legislation which limited the practice of medicine to registered doctors, that is, the products of orthodox medical schools. In turn, they themselves established a number of medical colleges, most of which were no more than diploma mills, where their graduates, in return for generous payment, received a very dubious MD qualification, but had in fact received little or no training. Such diploma mills exist to this day in that great land of free enterprise and initiative.

In the mid-years of the 19th century, medicine in the United States and to a somewhat lesser extent in Britain, was in a strange state of flux. The old Heroic Medicine was rejected by virtually all, physicians and patients alike. Proper and acceptable scientific research was proving the effectiveness of herbal medicine. But no scientific evidence was able to prove, or disprove, the effectiveness of homeopathy, and yet homeopathy was very obviously effective, and was shown to be so during the devastating epidemics of cholera which swept through the eastern United States. The homeopaths there, like their colleagues in Europe, treated their cholera patients with frequent and regular tiny doses of camphor, and it worked. It was easy and painless and cheap, unlike the unsuccessful efforts of the regular physicians. The patients of the Thomsonian practitioners and other herbalists did recover, but the treatment was at best uncomfortable, and demanded a lot of payment for repeated visits and quantities of medicine.

What was more, those homeopaths, who listened so carefully to their patients, were all fully qualified regular doctors. They became increasingly popular, and that growing popularity was matched by an increasing unpopularity of both regular medicine and Botanic medicine. The herbalists' treatment certainly worked, but was often unpleasant to endure.

The Eclectics met this problem head-on. They had already developed an impressive *materia medica*, which included new research on native American plants. A considerable botanical pharmaceutical industry was developing from which the Eclectics bought their medicines ready made. However, those 'crude and nauseating preparations' were beginning to lose their popularity. Was it possible, then, to extract from the crude herb all its active properties and discard what was inactive?

There was a subtle difference between what those chemists and scientists sought, and what the earlier chemists had produced. Earlier, the chemists had sought, and often found, one vital principle in a herb (like the diuretic principle of our old friend the dandelion): the Eclectic chemists would include not just the major active principle but all the other active ingredients that aided and modified the major action. Only the totally inactive parts of the herb would be discarded as useless dross. In many cases they succeeded in their search, and soon Concentrated Principles of various herbs appeared, and were immediately popular.

It all became a great bonanza for the pharmaceutical producers, for those handy herbal products were widely prescribed by the regular physicians as well as by the Botanic practitioners. The pharmaceutical industry flourished and became even richer.

Unfortunately, the Concentrated Principles were not particularly effective, as any old-time herbalist could have predicted. Even the most skilled and conscientious chemist could not unlock all of nature's secrets. They could not do that then: they cannot do it now. Many of the Eclectics reverted to producing their own medicines, as did those herbalists, in Britain and America, who had been seduced by the apparent simplicity of the Concentrated Principles.

Heroic Medicine was dead, finally killed off by the new generations of physicians revolted by the centuries of blood letting, mercury and purging. A new and kindly practice of medicine was required. Besides, it was becoming obvious that the physical make-up of people was declining. Army recruits were pathetically less robust than their forefathers had been, and women, in particular, seemed to be affected. That was hardly surprising, since women were subjected to treatment with mercury from childhood onwards. Blood letting and calomel were the solutions to all menstrual problems and to any problems of pregnancy. One of the worst results of dosing with calomel – which was mercury – was that it made the patient particularly susceptible to tuberculosis, and all of those pale, wan young women one meets repeatedly in Victorian fiction, spending their days reclining on a couch and suffering from 'a decline' were almost certainly tubercular, and were tubercular because of dosing with calomel.

The allopathic practitioners, the regular physicians, began using gentler, more kindly drugs, many of them plant based, and were the more successful in doing that. They adopted, and adapted, many of the principles of the Eclectics and eventually absorbed the Eclectics themselves, and that branch of healing in turn disappeared into the mists of history.

Meanwhile, the traditional herbalists continued on their way, many of them now boasting an MD degree from questionable American schools of medicine. In Britain, as in America, they had tried, and largely rejected, the Eclectic preparations, and soon reverted to the old and tried simple tinctures, teas, inhalations and ointments of their predecessors.

Again, the times were changing. The worst excesses of the early Industrial Revolution were over, and people had more, a little more, money to spend. Compulsory education was producing a society at least semi-literate, and news sheets and the soon-to-be ubiquitous bill board spread throughout Britain. Widely advertised patent medicines flooded on to the market, promising relief for every ill of humanity, from a headache to an unwanted pregnancy.

Improved sanitation in the towns and cities meant that many diseases virtually vanished, malaria and cholera amongst them, and they were the very diseases that herbal medicine treated so successfully. It seemed that the day of the traditional herbalist, with his jars of dried herbs and his bottles of unappetising tinctures, was finally over. But the practice of herbalism refused to die, although certainly it had to modernise. It was not enough any longer to know empirically that this condition responded well to that herb: it was becoming necessary to know why and how it responded, and also necessary to know what caused the symptom in the first place.

The British Reformed Medical Association had evolved into the National Association of Medical Herbalists, and that body was the voice of organised herbalism. The Association attempted to unite all irregular practitioners into one body which would be powerful enough to withstand the continued sniping and attacks of the allopathic practitioners and their repeated attempts to outlaw the unlicensed practice of medicine.

It began with wonderful efficiency and energy. John Skelton, in his sixties but still very active and vigorous, was one of the leaders, but even his enthusiasm and drive could not hold the Association together. The college they planned never materialised, and their regular magazine became thinner and finally withered away completely.

The new route that British herbalism had to take was well exemplified by Napiers of Edinburgh. This herbal practice and dispensary was established by Duncan Napier in Edinburgh in 1860. Duncan had no formal training and little formal education, but was a wonderful healer. His sons, and his grandson, who followed into the profession, were trained scientists who brought research and learning with them, to complement their perhaps innate healing skills. They needed those new skills if they were to function properly in a new era.

At one time sinking to as few as 90 members, the Association nevertheless continued to fight its corner, and was a constant irritant to the forces which attempted time and time again to outlaw herbalism. Most of the Association's time and energy was devoted to this cause, and even today the National Institute of Medical Herbalists – the direct off-spring of the Association – must still fight that war.

They set up training and educational schemes, and only those who had successfully completed arduous courses of study were admitted to membership. They rapidly became skilled at public relations and Parliamentary lobbying, and repeatedly defeated attempts to forbid the unlicensed practise of medicine.

Of course, they could not have succeeded in all of this without the support of very many people indeed. Although the country was flooded with patent medicines, there were still many places where the local herbalist was the only source of what was by now trained medical help. Time and time again, the herbalists sought to achieve recognition as Registered Practitioners, and repeatedly were refused.

Perhaps because the British public always has a strong regard for the under-dog, and certainly also because many in positions of power resented the arrogance of the medical professions in their incessant search for a monopoly of healing, herbalism not only refused to die, but in the early years of the 20th century began again to expand.

Meanwhile the profession of doctoring seemed to fall more and more into the financial hands of the drug companies. They financed the colleges, supported the journals, handed out endless samples of their products and entertained members of the profession at conferences which always seemed to be held in expensive hotels at attractive resorts. Of course, the vast amount of research being done did produce very powerful and effective remedies, which could be patented, then exploited, and publicised to the limit. The doctors could hardly be blamed for taking the easy way of prescribing: they remembered the (subsidised) article they had glanced at in the Journal, and its accompanying full-page advertisement. They remembered that happy week at the Conference in Florida. They checked blood pressure with an instrument bearing the name of the drug company. They wrote their prescription on a pad thoughtfully provided by the drug company with a pen also bearing its name. Even if they knew that in properly conducted trials garlic gave the best results as a treatment for tuberculosis, they still used the familiar drugs they had in fact been carefully conditioned to use.

Sarsaparilla (*smilax arnato*), for example, had first been introduced to Europe as a cure for syphilis. Whatever its success, it was soon replaced by the horrors of mercury treatment, but later careful studies showed that the simple sarsaparilla could help, even cure, syphilis patients who had gone through the courses of mercury and were so debilitated as a result that further treatment was inadvisable. Those patients responded well to large doses of sarsaparilla, but it never seemed to occur to the hospital doctors that they should try the herb in the early stages of the disease. The herbalists could not do that: they were forbidden by law from treating any venereal disease.

Herbalism refused to die. For whatever reasons, the sick turned again and again to herbal remedies, and to those who studied and prescribed them. That had been true for centuries, and it is still true today.

The qualified herbalist today, in Britain, is a highly trained professional, a skilled healer who seeks the cause of the symptom, and knows how to end it, and to cure the underlying disease.

Summing Up

> The Lord hath created medicines out of the earth, and he that is
> wise will not abhor them.

To sum up all of the above, we might begin by asking just what is a
herb? The dictionary says it is a plant the stem of which dies back
at the end of the growing season, and, secondly, an aromatic plant
used in cooking and medicine. The word comes from the Latin
herba, meaning grass or green plants. So a herb is a plant, and if we
look at plants in their world-wide context, we realise that without
plants, life on earth, including our life, would be impossible. We rely
on plants to trap the sole source of energy we have, that is, energy
from the sun. They trap that energy, convert it, and make it available to us, their fellow inhabitants of the earth. They produce most
of the oxygen on which we depend. They control the amount of car-
bon, water and hydrogen in the atmosphere.

That is what they do in the great picture of things, but looked
at individually, they perform even more incredible things. Each and
every plant in the world, from the humblest lichen to the greatest
forest tree, is a wonderful chemical factory. Out of nothing but sunlight, air, water and nutrients drawn from the soil, they produce
proteins, sugars, enzymes, hormones, oils and even pesticides.

Ultimately, all other organisms, including us, rely totally on
plants for our food. The sirloin steak we eat for dinner originated
in plants. The mouse that creeps through the grass on the lawn is
seeking plant seeds for its supper. The elephant, weary after a day
spent dragging huge logs out of the Asian forest, dines off a heap
of leaves and twigs.

All who practise herbal medicine are fully aware of this
remarkable relationship, a relationship which has existed, grown
and matured, since time immemorial. But it is with the wonderful
herbal chemical factory that herbal medicine is concerned.

We will never know – can never know – which of our primitive ancestors first noticed that eating a particular plant seemed to
cure a headache, or that certain cooling leaves seemed to make
wounds heal and bruises disappear. We do know that very far

back in human history our ancestors had considerable knowledge of the healing powers of plants. We have already noted that, four and a half thousand years ago, the Chinese scribe, Shen Nung, wrote the *Pen Ts'ao*, and this lists 364 plants used then in healing, and, remarkably, many of them are still used today.

So the medical herbalist today is not the cranky quack doctor so often derided by conventional doctors or ill-informed journalists. Rather she (and it is usually and traditionally 'she') is the modern depository of an ancient knowledge, used and tested by generation after generation, in a way that no product of a pharmaceutical factory can be. As the historian already quoted wrote, 'They (herbs) have been subjected to the longest clinical trial in history.'

Even today, according to the World Health Organisation, only 15% of the world's population have ready access to conventional (allopathic) medicine: the vast majority still rely on traditional healers, mostly herbalists.

Moreover, even in the most developed of countries, such as those of Western Europe and North America, herbal medicine, far from declining and dying, is alive and well and growing fast.

The reasons for this are many and complex, but basically it seems that there is a growing disquiet about the methods and results of allopathic medicine. In some fields, like surgery and the treatment of infections, modern medicine has undoubtedly made enormous progress. However, many chronic conditions like arthritis, eczema and heart disease grow more prevalent, and seem to threaten becoming pandemic. It is certainly not by the herbalist's choice that so many patients are suffering from long-standing chronic problems, who have all too often gone through perhaps years of medication and testing, to their frustration and to the frustration of their doctors. When finally the patient appears in the herbalist's consulting room, the problem is often tenacious, and the visit almost a cry of despair.

The practice of herbal medicine aims not only to bring relief from symptoms but to encourage an improved standard of general health and vitality. The diagnostic techniques of qualified herbalists resemble those of general practitioners, using the same equipment; but as well as assessing presenting symptoms, the practitioner looks beyond these to evaluate the over-all balance of the body's systems to discover underlying and predisposing disharmonies. Thus, entirely different remedies may be successfully given to treat two patients apparently suffering from the same complaint.

As well as examining the patient, the herbal practitioner will also want to discuss diet, exercise and lifestyle. Good nutrition is of vital importance: much of the food consumed today is refined, processed and preserved, with a resultant loss of original goodness, and contains many chemical additives. Many patients benefit almost immediately by changing to a properly balanced wholefood diet.

Whole plant remedies are ideally suited to this approach. Herbal practitioners disagree profoundly with the allopathic approach of finding, isolating and synthesising an active principle (e.g. aspirin from willow bark, quinine from cinchona bark, dioxin from foxglove, reserpine from rauwolfia, etc.) since the active isolated ingredients taken out of their herbal context are in the long term incompatible with good health. In plants, however, these powerful constituents are balanced, potentiated and made more or less accessible by numerous other constituents naturally present. The Chinese herb, ma huang (*Ephedra sinica*), for example, is invaluable in treating bronchial asthma, bronchitis and whooping cough. The chemists extract the drug ephedrine from the plant, and this is widely used to treat asthma and chronic bronchitis. However, ephedrine is an alkaloid which will raise blood pressure, and that must also then be treated. On the other hand, in the whole plant there are six other alkaloids, the main one of which actually prevents a rise in blood pressure and an increase in the heart rate. The isolated drug is dangerous, but the whole plant is balanced by Nature in such a fashion as to make it a much safer remedy.

Duncan Napier of Edinburgh, as a very young man, prepared a lobelia syrup, and cured his chronic cough. It was perhaps almost by accident that he used lobelia, but accident or not, he was using one of the most useful of all relaxants, with a profound depressant action on the nervous system and on neuro-muscular action – on coughing, in other words. More than that, though, one of the constituents, lobeline, is a powerful respiratory stimulant. Lobelia is a wonderful example of an holistic combination of relaxation and stimulation, and, properly used, has a profound effect on upper respiratory infection and bronchitis.

Herbal remedies do not have the aggressive and invasive action of modern drugs. Instead they provide the necessary trace elements, vitamins and medicinal substances in harmonious whole so as to return the patient to full health.

If you consult a qualified herbalist today, after the initial consultation (all consultations are in confidence), the patient's progress will be reviewed on subsequent visits and adjustments made to the herbal prescription as the practitioner then deems necessary. Herbal remedies are robust and effective and will often correct a problem quickly, but in chronic cases, the patient may need to take the remedies over a period of weeks or months, making such adjustments to diet and lifestyle as are necessary. In doing so, the patient and practitioner work together, partners in their common goal.

The herbal remedies prescribed may be indigenous, or they may have been imported from many other parts of the world. Harvesting, storage and processing are carried out to retain the optimum value of each remedy. Plant medicines are most commonly prescribed in liquid form as tinctures, fluid extracts or syrups, but may, on occasion, be given dried, to be taken as infusions or decoctions, or in powdered form as tablets or capsules. Local applications, ointments, lotions and poultices may also be prescribed as required.

When consulting a qualified Medical Herbalist (they will have the initials MNIMH or FNIMH behind their name) you will find a sympathetic and skilled practitioner, willing to give you time, care and natural remedies which offer a gentle yet effective way back to health.

In a consultation with a medical herbalist there will be no sense of haste or pressure. The consultation will last as long as necessary – thirty to forty-five minutes is normal – and the herbalist will enquire closely about diet, exercise and general lifestyle. The herbalist looks far beyond the symptoms of the illness and into the balance of the body's systems, seeking to discover all the underlying disharmonies which have led the body to rebel and to present the illness itself as a symptom of an underlying problem. Whilst of course seeking to alleviate the symptoms, the herbalist tries to cure the cause of the symptoms.

Almost certainly the patient will be given a prescription of herbs to take, but also almost certainly will receive advice on lifestyle and diet. Many patients benefit almost immediately on changing to a properly balanced diet of whole food, free, so far as possible, from the additives which contaminate so much of our refined, processed, preserved food. The prescription is likely to be for a tincture, a herbal extract. That tincture is prepared from the whole herb, and is not a single constituent, chemically extracted, but a combination of all the manifold trace elements, vitamins and medically active substances in one harmonious whole. Again, the aim is to treat the patient, and not just the illness.

So who and what is this herbal practitioner? And why is she or he qualified to treat illness? Most are young, and dedicated to their profession, and all have studied long and hard for their qualification. In Britain they have in fact studied for at least four years, either at the School of Phytotherapy, at the Scottish School of Herbal Medicine, or, more recently, at one of the British Universities which now offer degree courses in herbal medicine.

Much of the training is just the same as that taken in any medical school, except for surgery. A great deal of study is devoted entirely to herbs, their qualities, history and effects on the body. In the later years of study, hundreds of hours are devoted to clinical work where the student, under supervision, learns how to examine patients, take a history, and devise a suitable and effective course of treatment and prescription.

And then, after a stringent theoretical and practical final examination, the new herbalist can assume the title of Member of the National Institute of Medical Herbalists – MNIMH.

Herbal medicine is common to all races and peoples – Asian, Chinese, Egyptian, Greek, Roman, Indian and others. A Chinese herbal written in 2500 BC listed 365 herbs. Papyri from Egypt dated

1550 BC reveal a knowledge of 700 plant medicines, many of which are known and used today: elder, juniper, gentian, fennel, linseed, myrrh and peppermint among them.

During the Greek and Roman civilisations, Hippocrates, Galen, Dioscorides, Theophrastus and many other healers extended herbal knowledge, providing detailed medicinal and botanical descriptions. Following the advent of printing came many great European herbals, one of the most famous being *Gerard's Herbal*, printed in 1636, which gave the medicinal uses of very many plants.

This extraordinary history shows that the majority of herbal remedies in current use have been used for centuries or even thousands of years. The countless men, women and children who have had their health restored through the centuries by herbal remedies have proved their efficacy and safety in ways no modern clinical trial can emulate. Today, scientific research into the medicinal properties of various herbs is constantly being carried out, with results that frequently satisfy even the most stringent requirements of modern science. The National Institute of Medical Herbalists in Britain has its own research department which has contributed to the production of the *British Herbal Pharmacopoeia*, a work which covers the scientific description of medicinal plants used by British herbal practitioners.

Currently only comparatively few herbal remedies have been researched fully using our latest scientific methods. There are over three-quarters of a million species of plants awaiting investigation. Such is the bias of modern medicine that funds are rarely available for the verification and exploration of herbal remedies. Because a plant cannot be patented (unless of course it has been genetically modified) there is little incentive for expensive research, and what research is done is usually devoted to attempts at extracting an active constituent or principle from the whole plant, and that can be patented and exploited.

It is also worth noting that there is a tremendous interest these days in natural medicine and the use of herbs. One result of this is that every chemist's shop, health food store and even every corner shop has a shelf-full of 'herbal remedies'. Sadly, only too often these are adulterated and diluted almost beyond recognition. When you go to buy a herbal product, do try to get it from a herbal apothecary, where you can be sure of sound advice if you need it, and a product that is pure and fresh and effective.

PART II

Herbalism in Scotland

To Make Lilly of the Valley Water

Take the flowers OF the Lilly of the Valley and distil them in sack
and drink a spoonful or two as there is occasion. It restores
speech to those who have the dumb palsy. It is good against the
Gout; it comforts the heart and strengthens the memory; and the
flowers, put into a glasse, close stopped and set into ane hill of
ants for the month, then take it out and you find a liquor which
comes from the flowers, which keep in a vial; it is good, ill or
well, and whether man or woman.

Likewise for sprains, rub it in; and for the cholic, a great
spoonful in the hour.

THAT RECIPE FOR 'Lilly of the Valley Water' was one of the three gifts
young David Balfour carried as he left his childhood home to seek
his fortune. David Balfour was the central figure, although not the
hero, of Robert Louis Stevenson's novel *Kidnapped*. The gifts were a
silver shilling, a small bible – 'just big enough to fit into a plaid-neuk'
– and the recipe, and they were given to him by his minister.

The mention of this herbal remedy has always intrigued me.
Lily of the Valley is rare in Scotland, but was common in England
in the years that RLS was writing about. It was so common that it
had many different names, including Our Lady's Tears and Ladder
to Heaven. *Convalleria majalis*, to give its scientific name, was
highly regarded by both Gerard and Culpeper, and Lilly of the
Valley Water was held to be so precious that it was called *aqua
aurea*, or Golden Water, and those lucky enough to have some
were advised to keep it in vessels of gold or at least silver.

It is fascinating to speculate how RLS knew about this recipe.
Kidnapped was written in 1886, and by then Duncan Napier's
Herbal Dispensary and Clinic was flourishing in Edinburgh.

Robert was a sickly child, and grew up to be a sickly adult. His parents had travelled with the lad extensively in Europe, seeking a climate which might help him. Finally, he developed tuberculosis, which eventually killed him. I wonder if in his sickly childhood he had been treated with the very common mercury compound, calomel, a treatment which predisposed to tuberculosis. And had he perhaps also been treated with the kinder, gentle, herbal method of Duncan Napier?

Somehow he knew of Lilly of the Valley Water. Moreover, the recipe young David Balfour was given came from his minister, whose wife would doubtless have administered medication to the congregation, as all ministers' wives did in those days, so it is reasonable to assume that RLS knew of that practice.

We cannot know now, but it would not be surprising if the Stevenson family had been patients and customers of Duncan Napier. Certainly RLS himself must have been familiar with the old herbals, because the recipe he gives is very similar to that in the old books.

Even today, Lily of the Valley is a valuable herb used by herbalists in treating heart problems. It is a so-called Schedule Three Herb, held to be poisonous, and prescribed only by qualified herbalists.

Geologically, the Scotland we know today is a very young country, even though it contains some of the oldest rocks in the world. Around 300,000 years ago, land bridges connected what is now Scotland with the European mainland, and although there is no proof of this, it is reasonable to suppose that people migrated over those bridges from Europe. All evidence of that migration has long since vanished, ground to oblivion by the mile-thick glaciers of the Ice Ages, glaciers whose slow and inexorable progress also ground down the original mighty mountains into the majestic landscape we know today.

The last great glaciers retreated to the cold north about 10,000 years ago, leaving a strange land of bare rocks and mighty rivers. It was a new, virgin landscape, and one which very quickly became re-populated by various herbs, bushes and shrubby trees. Small animals followed, and then man re-appeared.

The earliest known settlement in Scotland is on the island of Rum. Dating back to 8,500 years ago, those Mesolithic or Middle Stone Age people were hunter-gatherers. We might legitimately call them scavengers. They lived off what they could find, living or dead, picking herbs in season, collecting seaweeds and shellfish from the shore, sheltering in caves or rock crevices. Naturally, they have left little evidence behind them: a few flint flakes where cutting tools have been chipped out of pebbles, and middens full of fish shells – mussels and oysters mostly. There seemed to be no animal husbandry or crop cultivation for another 4,000 years, although they did learn to hunt some of the larger animals, and thus obviously had learned to co-operate, since hunting and killing an elk cannot be done by one person.

The products of the land were their basic mainstay, and they learned to use plants in the most remarkable manner, not just as food, but as clothing, heating, bedding, weapons and implements. And, doubtless, as medicines.

In Scotland there is as yet no direct evidence of this wonderful sophistication in their use of plants, but a few years ago the Ice Man was disgorged from a glacier on the northern Italian border, and he came from the same period. Well preserved by his icy grave for 4,000 years, it is likely that he had perished in some winter's storm while travelling.

The Ice Man had been warmly clothed in woven grasses – although obviously not warm enough – and was equipped with a great variety of plant products, from a pack made of tree bark, to a bow and arrows of wood, dried moss for lighting a fire, plant fibres for bow strings and others at whose use we can only guess. In all, the Ice Man carried the products of sixteen species of plants and trees. Those people, wherever they were, clearly lived in harmony with their environment.

Slowly, as the generations passed, the people of Scotland progressed from hunting and scavenging to animal husbandry and cultivation. With that change came a more settled and regular diet which remained basically unchanged for the next 2,000 years, until about 300 years ago, when the potato was introduced. Before then, the only major change was the introduction of oats, which came to Britain with the Romans, and slowly spread north, to become a staple foodstuff for men in Scotland and for horses in England, as Samuel Johnson so memorably remarked.

Evidence from archaeological digs and pollen science show it to have been a healthy and varied diet, mostly vegetarian, and the wild product of the woods and hillsides as much as cultivated crops. Fruits and nuts, especially hazel nuts, acorns, and beech nuts, mushrooms, seaweeds, pig nuts and sow thistles were all used in season, plus cultivated turnips and swedes, with kale of various kinds, eggs, with fish and small game. Cattle were kept for milk and leather, and the milk was often made into butter and cheese. The cattle were too precious to be slaughtered for meat, although blood was often drawn from them to make what is still one of Scotland's favourites, black pudding.

A healthy diet, then, which produced a healthy people.

Scotland is a small country, and the Scots a small nation. Geographically, if not otherwise, firmly attached to the much bigger nation of England, much of Scottish history has been determined by that geographical propinquity, a propinquity popularly described as similar to being in bed with an elephant. That is as true today as at any time in written history. Whether it will remain so is not as clear.

That association had profound effects in all parts of Scotland's development, and not least in the development of healing, as we shall discover.

A small nation, yes (about five million today), and yet one divided into two parts in almost every conceivable way. Roughly speaking, those parts are the Highlands and the Lowlands. Strange as it seems, those familiar terms do not mean just that the Highlands are mountainous, and the Lowlands less high. The terms in fact reflect distance from the centre of government, and refer to different unrelated languages, Gaelic and Scottish, as well as, in recent centuries, to different religious affiliations and different loyalties.

Basically, the Highlands lie north of an imaginary line running south west to north east from the centre of the country. The Highlands are north of that line. Simplistically, the inhabitants were Gaelic speaking, Catholic, adherents of the Stuart crown, organised in the clan system, and far removed from the centres of political power, whether London or Edinburgh. The Lowlanders were none of these.

These differences led to profound differences in the development of healing. In truth, there is little difference between healing and its history in the Lowlands and that which took place in other adjacent areas of England. The influence of John Wesley was as great there as it was in the industrial towns of northern England. The Highlands in this, as in most things, were very different. It is that distinctive system which interests me most.

Until 300 years ago, the Highlands were hardly known to the rest of Britain, except as a distant, troublesome place, inhabited by a strange people, speaking a strange language, warlike, and as little known, it was said, as the cannibals of Borneo. They were believed to be painted savages, half naked in their tartan plaids, owing their primary allegiance to their clan chiefs, and paying little attention to the demands and laws emanating from either Edinburgh or London (an attitude still surprisingly strong within my own memory). They were thought of, in fact, as the Bravehearts of the day.

In other words, and more truthfully, they were an isolated but coherent society, virtually untouched by the ways and progress of the rest of the country.

This isolation was not necessarily by the choice of the people themselves, but it was imposed upon them by their clan chiefs and other feudal superiors, who carefully kept them separate from all the social and economic changes and progress taking part in the rest of Europe, including the Lowlands of Scotland. They were chattels, the property of their chiefs, who measured their wealth by the number of fighting men they could put into the field during the interminable clan wars of almost a thousand years.

This is all true enough, but like all generalisations, it is only half true. Certainly in terms of healing and healers, much that was ancient and unchanged remained pure and pristine there. The Highlanders were as self-contained in their healing as in their society as a whole. To understand how and why healing flourished for so long there, and left us such a legacy of knowledge, we need to understand that it was in reality a relic of social isolation.

Not, of course, that the kings and prelates and chiefs allowed themselves to be without the best of professional, trained medical help.

The family of Beatons, or MacBeths, were hereditary doctors, and from the early 14th to the late 16th century they attended to the health of Scottish lords and kings. The Beatons, although perhaps isolated from change themselves, were well equipped with the best of medieval medical knowledge. They possessed extensive libraries, containing the works of Avicenna, de Vigo, Gordonus and Hippocrates, and they practised according to the precepts of those great teachers. Not content with that, though, they had the practice of writing extensive marginal notes in their precious books, detailing how and why they treated the ills and wounds of their patients. Those books had probably come to them by way of Ireland, for the original Scots had come over the narrow sea from Ireland, bringing with them the Gaelic language of the Highlanders. Although equipped with a good knowledge of the late and mid-medieval tracts, those Beatons knew much more. Hector Boece, the 16th century Scottish historian and philosopher, attributed their success to 'their knowledge of the nature of every herb that grows in their country, and cures all manner of maladies therewith'.

As long ago as 1305, a Gaelic translation was made of *Lilium Medicinae*, written by Bernard Gordon, Professor of Medicine at the University of Montpellier. Several copies of this have survived, and it is said that one Beaton in Skye paid sixty milch cows for his copy. It was so precious to him that when he was visiting a patient and had to cross an arm of the sea, he would arrange to have his book carried round by land, rather than trusting it to the waters.

There are records of 76 individual Beaton physicians in late medieval Scotland, and records of the high esteem in which they were held. There is also a wealth of legends – or myths – of their successes. My own favourite is of the Beaton called to the bedside of a McLeod chief suffering, indeed dying, from an ulcer or growth in his throat which prevented him from speaking. Many other doctors had gathered to treat McLeod, but all had failed, for the ulcer was too deep in the man's throat to reach with a knife, and the knife was the only solution they could find.

Beaton examined his patient carefully, then asked that all the other doctors and attendants leave the room, leaving him alone with his patient. He then lifted his kilt, or dropped his trews, and made a large bowel movement on a convenient fire shovel. This he then placed on the fire to dry, and he and the astounded, but silent, McLeod waited until the contents of the shovel was dry and powdered. Letting this cool, Beaton then called back the doctors and attendants, and told them that this mysterious brown powder was the remedy he proposed to administer to McLeod.

They felt it, smelt it, looked closely, but could not determine what this mysterious substance was. They passed it around amongst themselves, finally each taking a pinch and trying it for taste.

This was too much for McLeod, who gave a great shout of laughter, the first sound he had been able to make for days, and laughed so much that the strain burst the ulcer and MacLeod recovered and suitably rewarded Dr. Beaton.

The Beatons are the best recorded of the hereditary Scottish physicians, but they were not the only ones. We also have good records of the McConachers of Lorne, and no doubt others will come to our knowledge as more ancient Gaelic manuscripts are deciphered.

The National Library of Scotland has in its collections a copy of a 15th or 16th century Gaelic manuscript, which is believed to have belonged to, and was perhaps written by, John Beaton. This, the *Regimen Sanitatis*, was indeed a Rule of Health. It includes many anecdotes and folk beliefs about health, and quotes other, much older, authorities. It emphasises, again and again, the importance of a sensible lifestyle, with moderation in eating and drinking, and taking much exercise.

On rising in the morning, the Gael was advised to stretch arms and chest, have a good clean spit and rub dust and sweat off his skin. He was to comb his hair, wash hands and face and clean his teeth. He should then pray, and exercise in high, clean places before breakfast. He was warned that great injury could be caused by raw things such as oysters, and by things half raw like birds badly roasted. (Shades of considerable outbreaks of illness recently in Scotland caused by just such things!)

Interestingly, whisky was often recommended, but usually flavoured with aromatic herbs such as mint, thyme, juniper and cranberry. Perhaps this was no more than a means of getting the patient to take the herb, a method similar to those still used by herbalists today (although not usually in whisky!)

The *Regimen Sanitatis* argued that there are three elements for the regulation of health. The first is guarding, the second foreseeing, and the third guiding backwards. The first means the maintenance of a state of health, which is the right of a healthy man. The second is the taking of the proper measures to remove the cause of the loss of health, and the third, which is a necessity, is the restoration of those who are ill.

The treatments used were an interesting combination of mystical and herbal techniques, and much use was made of water from particular magical or powerful wells. About 175 different herbs were used in ancient Gaelic medicine, most of them local, such as foxglove, broom, valerian and peppermint, but some were imported as spices, and it is presumed, although not yet proven, that these imports came through Ireland.

As well as medication, those healers, both the professionals like the Beatons and the unknown healers who treated their own families and neighbours, all used the power of magic wells, trees, stones and charms. Those wells were usually named after a saint, often Brigid, the goddess of healing. Their powers were limited: one cured madness, another scrofula and another fevers, and any ill-use of the well caused its spirit to desert that place and go elsewhere. Most areas of the Highlands have their own tales of the magic well and that it had 'always' been used with great success to cure madness, for instance. However, the tale often goes, one day a mad dog was taken and washed in the well, and although the dog was cured, the spirit of the well left in disgust, and never returned.

These beliefs lingered for centuries, and as the Highlanders grew less isolated, were the subject of much scorn from the orthodox medical men. But I wonder. Were the magic wells and stones and trees not a profound and skilful use of a placebo to cure a real

illness? Only today are we beginning to appreciate, if not understand, the remarkable powers of the placebo, in which some quite
inert substance, or some ritual, if used with authority and confidence by some respected figure, will often have a healing effect.
And it does not matter whether that figure of authority is a white-
coated doctor, a shaman dressed in feathers, or a wrinkled old
Wise Woman. I am very confident that the canny Highlander, over
many centuries, was not deceiving himself about those magic wells
and trees and stones. I am sure that they did produce results –
cures – and those cures were caused by a power which we might
call auto-suggestion, and which we are just now beginning to
investigate. Indeed, I suspect that the conventional medicine men
were moving along similar lines in their treatments. After all, they
were intelligent men, many of them, and it is at least possible that
their strange prescriptions, the donkey dung, stewed wood lice,
eye of toad and so on, as well as the incredible complication of
that universal panacea, theriac, were knowingly used as a placebo.

It is particularly interesting to me that in more than one of
those old Gaelic manuscripts there is reference to a cause of illness
being 'things small, minute, full of spite, venom and hostility' – a
vivid description of microbes!

There is little doubt that the feudal superiors had access to
professional medical help, but equally there is no doubt that the
mass of people did not. They were left to their own resources, and
those resources were considerable. Self-help was not a choice, but
a necessity, and a great mass of knowledge about plant healing
developed, and was passed on through generations of women.
Women, as always, were the healers, the nurses, the midwives, the
Wise Women, the howdies, the hen-wives. Men, on the other
hand, cared for the wounds of war, the broken and dislocated
limbs, and whatever surgery was attempted. And that primitive
surgery, even as long ago as The Late Stone Age, included the
strange operation of trepanning, in which a disc of bone is cut out
of the patient's skull, for what purpose we really do not know –
perhaps to release evil spirits, or perhaps to relieve headaches.
Several such trepanned skulls have been found in Scotland, and
many in other countries, and obviously the operation was suc-

cessful, in so far as the patient did not die, for their wounds healed, and they lived long after the operation, whether restored to health or not we cannot know.

Not that women were always left in peace to practice their healing art. For centuries the danger of being accused of witchcraft and sorcery hung over them. Witchcraft was recognised and accepted as a threat to Christianity, both Catholic and later after the Reformation, and only too often accusations of witchcraft were made against women who used herbs or other methods to treat disease. After all, the accepted Pauline version of Christianity saw only evil and temptation in women.

Happily, neither Scotland nor England suffered as much as some other European countries from the horror of the medieval witch-hunts. However, with King James VI – later James I of England – that all changed. James, the Wisest Fool in Christendom, was an educated man. He would have agreed with his contemporary Robert Burton, that great theologian, who wrote that 'witches steal young children out of their cradles and put deformed in their rooms, which we call changelings'. He would also have agreed with another contemporary, Thomas Browne the theologian, who wrote that 'I have ever believed, and do now know, that there are witches.'

It is easy to see why James believed these things. After all, he was convinced that he had had personal experience of the malevolence of witches. The King was enamoured with the idea of marrying Princess Anne of Denmark. It would, he was sure, be a good marriage, and would unite two dynasties. James sent an ambassador to Denmark, and, suitable arrangements having been made for dowries and alliances, the two were married by proxy, and the Princess sailed for Scotland. However, the convoy met repeated storms, and was driven to take shelter in a Norwegian fjord. The Danish admiral wrote that he was convinced that witches had raised the storms.

James decided to sail himself to fetch his bride. After a very stormy passage his ships reached Oslo, and the two were remarried. They stayed in Oslo for six months on an extended honeymoon, and then sailed for Scotland. Again gales struck the little convoy, and James became convinced that his own ship was subject to the particular malevolence of the elements. Surely, then, the Danish admiral was right in believing witchcraft was at its evil work. On reaching Scotland safely, James set up an investigation into his suspicions, and of course he was proved to be right.

There had indeed been a witches' gathering at North Berwick, and more than 100 people were involved, including six men. They had called on the Devil himself to prevent James from returning to Scotland. They had used spells and melted wax dolls. Finally they had raised the great storms by swinging cats three times widdershins (anti-clockwise) round their heads and hurling them into the sea. All this they confessed, after undergoing the most extreme tortures, even if one man, a school master, had retracted his confession. So they must all die in agony, and perhaps the Lord would receive their souls, although more likely those souls would join the Fallen Angel in the hellish depths below.

So James had been right, and he wrote a book about it. *Daemonologie* he called it, and liked it so much that when he became king of England as well as Scotland, had it republished in 1603 in London. It was a successful, popular and influential book, and initiated a witch hunt in Britain that led to the accusation, torture, confession and dreadful execution of over a thousand people, men and women.

Later, in Scotland during the Rule of Saints, when the Kirk controlled the State, 300 women were burned as witches in 1661-2, many of them accused of such heinous offences as giving a woman herbs to relieve the pains of childbirth. 'In sorrow shalt thou bring forth children' the Bible stipulated: to ease the pains was against the will of God, and could only have been done with the help of the Devil.

Fortunately the Highlands escaped much of this terror. It was the law that all legal processes (and the torture and burning of witches was legal) had to be confirmed in Edinburgh and be in English. The Highlanders used and understood only Gaelic, and it was just too much trouble and expense to have it all translated and sent to Edinburgh.

There is little amusing in all that horror, but we may be

allowed a small smile at what happened in 1552. John Hamilton, Archbishop of St. Andrews, was brought low again by his severe asthma. Doctors failed to cure him, although they tried all the strongest medicines in their repertoire. A travelling Italian Herb Doctor prescribed remedies, after studying the Archbishop for a long time. The sick man was advised to take coltsfoot and other herbs, to use kelp in his pillow and not feathers, and to have a sparse diet. He, the supposedly celibate Archbishop, was also advised to give up his practice of having sex every day before and after supper. John Hamilton was cured of his asthma (probably the main reason was giving up his feather pillow), but the good Dr Candora was accused of witchcraft, and narrowly escaped with his life.

A woman who successfully treated an earlier Archbishop of St Andrews was not so lucky. Alison Pierson, a gifted healer, cured the Archbishop of an illness that had defied his doctors. Far from being grateful, the Archbishop promptly accused Alison of witchcraft, supervised her torture, heard her confess, and watched her burn. Clearly, it was argued, if trained and educated men could not cure a disease, then that disease must be the result of witchcraft, and thus only someone in a compact with the Devil could remove it.

The Physicians argued otherwise, although the result was the same. Illness must be the will of God: surely then it could not be removed by any woman, for women were the daughters of Eve, who was directly responsible for the expulsion of man from the Garden of Eden. If she did indeed cure, then it must be by Devilish means. The result for the woman was the same – being handed over to the torturers and executioners for rape and torment and a slow agonising death.

There is a strange and rather ambiguous memorial to those supposed witches hard by the Edinburgh Castle Esplanade, the site where so many women died in the flames from the 16th to the early 18th century. This is a drinking fountain of bronze, now disused, in the Art Nouveau style, erected in 1894. It has a relief of 'witches' heads encircled and entwined by a snake (shades of the Garden of Eden!). A plaque explains that 'The wicked head and the serene head signify that some used their exceptional knowledge for evil purposes while others were misunderstood and wished their kind nothing but good. The serpent has the dual significance of evil and of wisdom. The foxglove sprig further emphasises the dual purpose of many common objects.' There is an Evil Eye portrayed, as well as the Hands of Healing. It is difficult to know just what message is conveyed by this plaque, but the implication seems to be that witches did exist, had particular powers, and that some at least of those powers were used for evil purposes. It was on that site that the last alleged witch died in the flames.

Perhaps the best and most complete description of medicine and healing in the 17th century Highlands comes from Martin Martin, a Lowlander who had studied medicine in the great school at Leiden in Holland. He travelled extensively through the Highlands and Islands, and wrote very entertainingly of his travels. He reported that the chief problems were 'fevers, stitches, cholick, headache, megrim, jaundice, sciatica, stone, small pox, measles, rickets, scurvy, worms, fluxes (diarrhoea), toothache, cough and squinance (tonsillitis)'. Martin describes the use of herbs, used internally and externally, ointments and plasters in treating what is, to us, largely a list of symptoms, rather than diseases.

How widely that healing knowledge was spread we cannot really tell today, but much of it is still recollected in the memories of old people. Nor, indeed do we know how many herbs, used in the day of Martin Martin, have ceased to grow in the Highlands as a result of the omnivorous grazing by the alien sheep introduced when the ancient clan system was finally broken after the last futile Jacobite rebellion of 1745. That was when Prince Charles Edward – Bonnie Prince Charlie – made his attempt to recover the throne of England and Scotland for the Stuart line. That rebellion, chiefly but not exclusively, a rebellion by Highlanders, led inexorably to the clearances, that time of appalling ethnic cleansing which resulted in the vast Diaspora of Highland folk to the colonies, and resulted also in the vast emptiness which is still the Highlands of Scotland.

Those cleared people took with them all their knowledge of healing, to the great benefit of the lands they settled. And that knowledge must have been considerable, because in spite of all the

hardships of life as peasants, and even after the horrors of the aftermath of the 1745 rebellion, it seems that the Highlander was generally a healthy specimen. Indeed, there is an ancient Gaelic proverb:
Is e an orighreachd an t-slainte – Health is the inheritance – which
suggests that the Gael expected to be healthy and regarded health as
a birthright. This, of course, was without the attention of trained
doctors. Or perhaps it was because there were no doctors.

In 1791, the first volume of a massive *Statistical Account of
Scotland* appeared. Eventually filling twenty large books, this was
initiated by the remarkable Sir John Sinclair, an agriculturist and
statistician. He persuaded the ministers of every parish in Scotland
to survey their parishes and report their findings. Housing, agriculture, health, population and occupations were all covered, and
the results were, and remain, an invaluable source of information..
The ministers reported: 'We have commonly no sickness.' 'Very
few diseases are known among the people.' 'Inhabitants are all
healthy.' 'No disease is peculiar to the parish from climate or any
other cause.' 'The people have very few diseases.' These were typical reports from the ministers.

It is reasonable, of course, to suppose that the ministers put
the best possible gloss on the state of their parishioners. Another
point of view was expressed by Donald MacLeod in his book
Gloomy Memories, a contemporary account, by one who suffered
them, of the Highland Clearances. Donald wrote that, after the
Clearances in various areas, and after the trauma of the 1745
rebellion and its hideous aftermath of slaughter, 'many severe diseases made their appearance, such as had hitherto been almost
unknown amongst the Highland population, viz. typhus fever,
consumption, and pulmonary complaints in all their varieties,
bloody flux, bowel complaints, eruptions, piles and maladies
peculiar to women.'

After the crushing of the 1745 rebellion and its awful aftermath, the power and laws of London and Edinburgh were spread
to the Highlands. Clan organisation and practices were declared
illegal, and although not expressly forbidden (as were wearing the
kilt and playing bagpipes, for example) herbal medicine found
itself under attack from another quarter.

The new lairds, priests and teachers imported to 'civilise' the Highlands and the Highlanders brought with them new medicines. Usually equipped with a medicine chest and a book of instructions, this new upper class proceeded to treat the deserving poor. Since their medicine chests typically contained little beyond senna pods, cascara tablets and bi-carbonate of soda, with Dover's Powder if they were really up-to-date, the good they could do was strictly limited. However, they represented the new, the powerful, the exotic, and quite clearly their ways must be best.

However, it seems that not all the poor were treated by the lairds and their ladies. In her *Memoirs of a Highland Lady*, Elizabeth Grant of Rothiemurchas noted that when a doctor was needed for one of the family, he had to be brought at great expense from a distant town. 'Medical aid', she wrote, 'being little wanted. Herbs and such simples cured the generality, and we had my grandfather's medicine chest administered very sagaciously by my father.'

Oddly, in the Lowlands, it was often the ministers who did the doctoring, and they seemed to delight especially in bloodletting and vaccination against smallpox. Just before service on each Sunday was the favoured time for this.

Remember that the mass of people, the young and strong, had been removed from their native land and transported to Nova Scotia, Virginia, Tasmania and New Zealand. Those left behind were not strong enough to resist new ways.

Especially in the Highlands, even the language of those new-come upper classes was exotic, for they spoke English and the Highlanders spoke and understood only Gaelic. Even in the Lowlands, understanding was difficult, for in those days the Lowland people still used Scottish exclusively, and although English and Scottish are related, they are not the same.

However, those imposed over us must be obeyed, and gradually it became accepted that it was better to have a dose of Epsom salts from the bountiful hand of the Laird's Lady than be attended to by 'the auld wifie doon the road', however much your parents had told you about her healing skills and successes.

Almost simultaneously with the Highland Clearances came the beginning of the industrial revolution. Much of Lowland Scotland became a vast industrial centre, the biggest in Britain and one of the biggest in the world. Coal mines, iron and steel factories, shipyards, ceramic works, locomotive building – virtually every aspect of industrial activity was founded and boomed there.

This brought great social changes. The factories demanded not just the raw materials to be converted into goods and of course profit, but also vast numbers of people to be converted into industrial workers, converted, mostly, from peasant farmers into an industrial working class. Many thousands of Scots, both Lowlanders and Highlanders, were cleared from the land, and guided, manoeuvred and forced into the new factories and mines. That process was assisted also by the agricultural revolution and new farming practices which meant that fewer farm workers were needed. And even then it was not enough. Thousands more families came from Ireland, bringing with them a different religion and different social organisations, some of which still trouble Scotland to this day.

Of course, the healing knowledge of the old times came with the people. But how could it be used? A Wise Woman who needed yarrow, larch and coltsfoot to treat the whooping cough (the rightly dreaded 'kinkcough' of the slums) in her child or the child of a neighbour certainly could not find the herbs in the awful stews where those industrial workers existed, and certainly she could not go back to her native Glencoe to get them.

Slowly but surely the traditional knowledge died in the factory towns as well as in the glens and straths of the Highlands. Some cures were still available. Potato, carrot and turnip were all often used as poultices, as were chopped leek, chewed tobacco and soap. Basically, though, the role of women in healing was reduced to attending childbirth, and that of men to bonesetting.

The history of our traditional healers has been neglected, although in my view such studies would cast much light into dark corners of our history. One who did some such studies was Dr. David Rorie, a GP who practised mostly in the coal mining areas of Fife. He is best remembered today as a collector of folk traditions and songs. He was himself a good poet and song writer, as well as a very brave man who was gratefully remembered by many after the hell of the Great War. In his studies of folk medicine, however, there is very little mention of herbal medicine.

Bonesetters loom large in his recollections and are the subject of much scorn and disdain. Spells, healing wells and healing trees are described at length, and dismissed as nonsense. The old placebos of carrying a potato to avoid rheumatism, or wearing a copper bracelet to avoid strains and sprains, and many more such are recorded. But not, strangely, herbal treatments.

This cannot be because he never met them. Can it be, then, that the good doctor was afraid of herbalism, seeing it as a threat to his own omnipotence and omniscience as a doctor? After all, if a Spey Wife – a traditional healer – could affect cures which were beyond his powers, and which he could neither understand nor explain, he was likely to be wary of attacking those cures.

Obviously, Dr. Rorie felt free to attack the bonesetters. Those men (always men) were dealing with the skeleton, something he knew well, and no doubt often enough they did fail to effect a cure. They often did cure, though, as I know well. As a lad I dislocated an elbow, and the police surgeon, after three painful attempts, had failed to reduce it. A man in a neighbouring village, a man who was 'skeely wi' banes' did the job, still in his work clothes and black from the pit. And, in the ancient tradition of healers, no money changed hands for the successful treatment.

Another story is illustrative of how traditional knowledge lingered on. My father was a village policeman in a coal-mining area. His job, his livelihood and that of his family, depended on his ability to walk miles of patrols, day and night. When rheumatism began to affect him, I was frequently sent out to gather nettles, not young and tender ones, but tough old stems. With these, my father proceeded to thrash his bare legs until they were red and the floor littered with leaves. He claimed that that traditional treatment, which he had learned from his grandfather, not only kept his rheumatism at bay, but actually cured it.

Interestingly, much of the tradition of folk medicine has been best preserved and remembered by the travelling folk, the Summer Walkers, who have been part of the Scottish scene for many centuries. They are itinerant workers who traditionally travelled the roads every summer, working at harvesting, tin-smithing, and selling the wooden implements and tools they spent the winter making. Those people, who are few and threatened today, have proved to be a vast reservoir of traditional beliefs, practices, songs, music and healing. In an interview one traveller, Essie Stewart, said: 'Mare's milk – being forced to drink mare's milk as a cure for whooping cough ...that's the first thing I remember. It was thin, very thin, like skimmed milk, sweet tasting. You have to drink it warm, straight from the pail. My mother dipped a tin cup and made me drink. It was frothy, almost yellow-gold.'

What was the situation of the unhappy masses in the growing towns? In Edinburgh the situation was appalling, and in Glasgow simply incredible.

Edinburgh, in fact, was two towns in those days, and indeed still is in many ways. The New Town, with its delightful crescents, squares and avenues of pleasing Georgian design, was increasingly prosperous and powerful in trade, finance, the law and theology. The Old Town, that romantic area around the beloved Royal Mile, was as crowded and degrading as anywhere in Britain.

A Medical Gentleman, writing of life in Edinburgh in mid-Victorian times, said:

> Around the castle in the wynds, closes and vennels of High Street and Canongate, Saturday night presents one of the most revolting sights ever witnessed. The filth, degradation and hopelessness is awful and could not be exceeded, indeed it may be gravely questioned if in any city in one night of the week, destitution, prostitution and crime ever held such review as they hold in the High Street of the modern Athens.

There were hospitals and dispensaries available for the poor, but even the poor had to pay, and often enough the poor could not pay. Then they must rely on the benevolent generosity and charity of the middle classes, and that was not always forthcoming, especially for those who were not properly grateful.

Records of Edinburgh's Royal Infirmary indicate that often patients were suffering from nothing but hunger, and they were kept in the hospital long enough for the good diet to produce the expected benefits.

It would be wrong, however, to think that the medical élite of Edinburgh, with their armoury of mercury, leeches, theriac and other appalling compounds, had altogether forgotten or forsaken their herbal roots. Sir Robert Sibbald, for example, encouraged as much as possible the use and study of herbs. It was he who was responsible for the establishment of Edinburgh's Botanical Garden, at first on a site now covered by Waverley railway station. It was the second Botanical Garden in Britain, and at first was devoted solely to growing and studying herbs for medical purposes. Later the Garden was moved to its present site, and became, what it remains to this day, the beloved 'Botanics', a delightful open space, in the middle of a great city. Much botanical and herbal research continues to be done there.

Sir Robert Sibbald produced *The Edinburgh Pharmacopoeia* in 1669, a listing and description of the plants growing in the Botanical Garden. Sir Robert also tried to show how Scotland could avoid another great famine such as that of the late 17th century, when crop failures led to the population dropping by 15% in five years. He advocated that the Scots should make use of the many native foods that were available, free and in plenty, but were not used. He listed otters, moles, stoats, squirrels and frogs. I greatly doubt that many conservative Scots followed that advice. However, Sibbald's argument in favour of kitchen gardens was certainly listened to, and those who had, or could get, a bit of land became keen gardeners, a tradition still present today, even if there are more dahlias grown than leeks nowadays.

The Edinburgh Medical School, founded in the early 18th century, was the first in a British University, and produced many very fine doctors. But this only affected a very few people – the rich and their households, and city dwellers who could gain admission to a hospital or could find a medical man to treat them at little or no cost. And many doctors did that, but the demand was much greater than the supply, and villages and even large towns often had no medical man available. In the mid-18th century, there was one doctor in Sutherland to cover 2000 sq. miles of the wildest country in Britain.

Thus, although traditional or folk medicine was central to the lives and deaths of 90% of Scots, little was available, especially in such centres as Edinburgh and Glasgow. It was in the slums of the industrial centres that medical help of any kind was most needed. Existing on a diet of adulterated flour, rotting meat, watered milk, mouldy cheese, stale fish and sprouting potatoes, the health of the people was appalling, and expectancy of life short. Only gin and illicit whisky and sex made life worth living.

In the countryside, by contrast, for those with access to a little land, as all farmworkers had, the diet was varied and healthy. Much of it could be gathered from hills and hedgerows: it did not even need cultivation. There was water cress, sloes, hips, raspberries, strawberries, earth nuts, seaweed, nettles, wild spinach, wild garlic and wild carrots – all consumed with enthusiasm by the country dweller of the 17th and 18th centuries, together, of course, with the ubiquitous oatmeal porridge.

It was in the empty spaces of the Highlands and the small villages there that the memory and practice of herbalism and other traditional healing lingered. In truth, there was no alternative: there simply were no medical men available, and who could afford them anyway? So you had to turn to the Wise Woman who lived down the road. Somehow, she retained some of the accumulated wisdom of centuries of healing. Somehow her female ancestors had escaped being burned at the stake, at the instigation of the Church, as witches, or at least had survived long enough to pass on their knowledge to another generation of Wise Women. Folk or Domestic Medicine had for many centuries been a necessary tool for survival, as it still is in many countries. Built up over the generations, and passed from generation to generation, it was the distilled wisdom of the ages. We are the poorer for its loss.

In the industrial cities, there was very little scope for herbal treatments. Even if the knowledge was there, the herbs were not. And yet it was in the cities that modern herbalism developed, amongst that great bubbling cauldron of dire poverty, immense wealth, dehumanising conditions and great elegance.

Amongst that great flowering of intellectual activity and new ideas which we call the Scottish Enlightenment, physicians began, in some cases, to question some of their ancient, well-loved precepts. One such was Dr. William Buchan, a graduate of Edinburgh, who in 1769 published his book *Domestic Medicine*.

Dr. Buchan was that medical rarity, a trained physician who questioned the wisdom of his teachers. He wrote that it was a characteristic of those who followed the 'trade' of medicine to have implicit faith in what they were taught and a devout attachment to established forms. And he called it a trade, not an art or a science. In his view the administration of medicines was always doubtful and often dangerous, and that was certainly true of many medicines then being being prescribed by the 'trade'. He believed it better to teach how to avoid the necessity of medicine than how to use it. Diet, hygiene and cleanliness were his major prescriptions, and simple herbal remedies if necessary.

Domestic Medicine was an immediate success, and ran to 22 editions. Together with the Good Book – the Bible – it could be found in virtually every cottage, in the Highlands as well as the Lowlands, and in the Lowlands there would also probably be a copy of Robert Burns's poems.

There are in fact clear resonances between *Domestic Medicine* and the ideas of good health and diet stipulated in the old clan physicians' writings, the Beatons and others. Sensible clothing and sensible food in moderation, exercise, cleanliness and clean water were, Dr. Buchan believed, essential. His advice to parents is as relevant today as it was 200 years ago. Children should be kept clean and their clothes changed as often as possible. Fathers should take a greater interest in the bringing up of their offspring, and when remedies were required, the common herbs were infinitely preferable to the compounded messes of the doctors and apothecaries. Dr. Buchan was also an early medical advocate of vaccination, used against smallpox, and this in particular roused the ire of his medical colleagues.

The runaway success of his book was well remarked by the powers in the land, and when he died he was accorded the singular honour, for a common physician, of being buried in Westminster Abbey, no doubt to the chagrin of his more illustrious medical colleagues.

Mid-Victorian Scotland

It was the best of times; it was the worst of times; it was the age of wisdom; it was the age of foolishness; it was the epoch of belief; it was the epoch of incredulity; it was the season of Light; it was the season of Darkness; it was the spring of Hope; it was the winter of Despair; we had everything before us; we had nothing before us; we were all going direct to Heaven; we were all going direct the other way...

When he wrote that first sentence of *A Tale of Two Cities*, Charles Dickens was referring to England and France in 1775: no-one, though, could have penned a better description of mid-Victorian Scotland, the time and place where Duncan Napier established his shop and practice.

By the middle of the 19th century, the population was growing fast. However, it was a population on the move. Scotland had been a country largely of agricultural workers, peasant farmers, crofters and home industries such as hand loom weaving and spinning; it was fast becoming a country of heavy industry and big cities.

Largely, though not entirely, concentrated in Scotland's Central Belt, between Edinburgh and Glasgow, those industries had an insatiable demand for labour. Men, women and children were needed for the mills, mines and factories, and they flocked there in their thousands. The Industrial Revolution produced an entirely new class of people, an industrial proletariat, who owned literally nothing but their strength and whatever skills they had managed to acquire.

They owned no land; they had been cleared or dispossessed. Their hand looms and spinning wheels were out-dated and broken up. Their cottages had been destroyed and the roof-timbers (their most valuable possessions) burned. Their cattle and their seedcorn had been eaten or wantonly destroyed on the orders of the landowners and their factors. Their clan chiefs and ministers of religion had deserted and forsaken them. They were destitute and desperate. Others, mainly from the Lowlands, had been agricultural workers and smallholders displaced by the enclosures of the Agricultural Revolution, with its consequent reduction in the numbers of farmworkers.

Robert Burns, as ever, had a word to say about this, and his poem *Man was made to Mourn – A Dirge* was probably the first poem about the sheer despair which afflicted those victims of the early Industrial Revolution.

> ...See yonder poor o'erlaboured wight,
>   So abject, mean and vile,
> Who begs a brother of the earth
>   To give him leave to toil;
> And see his lordly fellow-worm
>   The poor petition spurn,
> Unmindful, though a weeping wife
>   And helpless offspring mourn.
>
> If I'm designed yon lordling's slave,
>   By Nature's law design'd,
> Why was an independent wish
>   E'er planted in my mind?
> If not, why am I subject to
>   His cruelty or scorn?
> Or why has man the will and pow'r
>   To make his fellow mourn?
>
> ...O Death! The poor man's dearest friend,
>   The kindest and the best!
> Welcome the hour my aged limbs
>   Are laid with thee at rest!
> The great, the wealthy fear thy blow,
>   From pomp and pleasure torn;
> But, oh! a blest relief for those
>   That weary-laden mourn!

Scotland had been a nation of peasant farmers, in so far as it still remained a nation. In just a few years it was supplying much of the world with steel, ships, jute products, tweed and the produce of improved farming.

Great industrial progress, and the accumulation of immense wealth, was accompanied by, and even dependent upon, quite appalling social deprivation, misery and degradation. This small country, with its great and well-earned reputation for high thinking and a rigid morality, was built upon a foundation of almost indescribable squalor, of drink abuse, stinking housing, inadequate wages, impossibly long hours of labour, mal-nourishment and ill-health.

Today, we find it difficult to even envisage the life of a city carter, for example, with his 90-hour working week, outside in all weathers, and poorly clad against that weather. His only prospect was unending labour and an early death. His horse could at least look forward at the end of its working day to being dried off, fed, and given a bed of straw: the carter looked forward only to a walk home through the rain, a meal of potatoes, and a few hours sleep on a bed of rags. The horse and cart belonged to the man's employer and were valuable. The carter himself owned nothing but his physical strength and the ability to reproduce another generation of wage slaves.

Some few recruits to this strange raggle-taggle army did manage to escape the worst of the battle. They were the men – never the women – who acquired skills, the tradesmen and artisans. Their wages were better, their hours less, and their prospects somewhat less drear. They themselves possessed the tools of their trade and the skills to use them. They were the Aristocrats of Labour, the men who built the magnificent edifices of the mid-Victorian cities, who drove the locomotives and fashioned the steel of the ships.

They were the elders of the Kirk, the vocal advocates of temperance, the organisers of Trade Associations and primitive unions, the establishers of Co-Operative Societies. They were also, of course, the politically aware, the Chartists, for example, who were seen as threats to the stability of society and the economy.

However, when, as happened repeatedly, trade took a downturn, they had no more protection than the mass of unskilled workers. Indeed, in a sense, they could be worse off, since they had more to lose, and at least had had a glimpse of the possibility of a better life.

The honest working man was assured that life could be better and prospects bright. In his *A Century of the Scottish People, 1830 – 1950*, TC Smout quotes one such assurance. In 1849, the Rev. Blaikie of Pilrig Free Church, delivered *Six Lectures Addressed to the Working Classes*. Amongst much else, and most of it equally moronic, he said:

> Working people are sometimes apt to envy capitalists and to speak very bitterly against them, as if they sinfully monopolised the comforts of life. But in what way have capitalists obtained their capital? Very generally by the plan now described. Industry, patience, self-denial, abstinence from expensive habits and indulgences, delay in entering on the matrimonial state, and other such means, have enabled them to accumulate a capital which has grown by degrees to gigantic dimensions. We know of several cases in point. The way is open for others to go and do likewise.

This was a very typical middle-class attitude, and one which was shared by the City Fathers, many of whom were themselves landlords and builders. They believed, or at least argued, that there were two types of poor people, the respectable and the unrespectable, the deserving and the undeserving. It was the latter who had housing problems, and those problems were recognised. However, it was held that, basically, they were responsible for their own abject poverty. 'The root of the evil in the housing of the poor is the thriftlessness, intemperance and want of self-respect of a considerable class among tenant occupants.' But it would be an offence against the laws of nature and economics to intervene and make improvements: indeed, any interference with the market, whether in housing or international trade, was wrong by its very nature. Yes, it was agreed that there was poverty, but personal philanthropy and the charity of the churches should be left to deal with that, for they could distinguish between the deserving and the undeserving, and would not encourage the indigent or undermine the vital principle of self-help.

The present writer is no historian, and is certainly not equipped to present a study of those days, nor of the circumstances of those who endured them. However, many others are so equipped and have done so. Some brief quotations from contemporary sources are not out of place.

Since this book is about Napiers of Edinburgh, it is reasonable to ask what sort of place it was in those days, only 140 years ago, when Duncan Napier was studying his herbs, delivering his bread rolls and planning to open his shop.

Dr. Johnson wrote in 1775 that Edinburgh was even then 'A city too well known to admit description', but that has not deterred a thousand writers from doing so since then. The city is of course the capital of Scotland, built on a dramatic hilly site overlooking, and thus controlling, the Firth of Forth. The drama of the site was established about 325 million years ago, when the great Edinburgh Volcano, whose remnants we know as Castle Hill and Arthur's Seat, erupted and poured great streams of lava down its slopes.

Many millennia later, the great glaciers of the Ice Age met the immovable rock, and split into two main streams, gouging out deep hollows round the crags. The Grassmarket, the Cowgate and the Nor Loch (now Princes Street Gardens) were the result.

The first people appeared perhaps 7,000 years ago, and the crags and hills have been continuously occupied since then. The capital of a nation it may have been, the seat of the Crown and the centre of government, but it grew very slowly. By the end of the 14th century, it had only about 350 houses, and perhaps 2,000 inhabitants. In fact, it lay too near the border with England, the Auld Enemy, to grow in peace. Repeatedly, the township was attacked and occupied, especially during the Wars of Independence, when Scotland sought to assert freedom from attempted domination by the English.

Defensive walls were built, although they never quite encircled the town – defence to the north was provided by the Nor Loch. The Flodden Wall, built after the tragedy of Flodden Field, certainly provided a defence, but also provided a girdle beyond which the town could not safely grow. So since it could not grow outwards, it had to grow upwards. The Old Town of Edinburgh, with its 'slit-canyons, closes, courts and tenements' developed into what was surely the first 'High Rise' architecture, with some of the tenements reaching to as many as fourteen storeys.

Of course, it could not last. Expansion was essential. The Wars of Independence had been fought – and won – but the eventual Union with England was inevitable. The growth of trade, commerce and industry produced pressures which eventually burst the bounds of the City Walls, and Edinburgh New Town began to grow on the opposite side of the Nor Loch, that stinking swamp and sewer.

In 1752 the Convention of Royal Burghs agreed on 'Proposals for Carrying out Certain Public Works in the City of Edinburgh'. They resolved 'Let us enlarge Edinburgh to the utmost.' And this they did. An elegantly simple grid plan put forward by James Craig was accepted and the 'Athens of The North' began to take the shape we know and love today.

The merchants, manufacturers and professional people migrated *en masse* to the gracious squares and crescents, leaving the strange hugger-mugger of the Old Town to the poorer people. No more did the old tenement buildings house the upper and the middle classes in the first two or three storeys with the poorer people high above.

From then on, and still today, there are in reality two Edinburghs. 'Spatial segregation of the social classes' had been declared to be civic policy: it sometimes seems still to be so.

In 1861, the population of Scotland was 3,062,294, according to the census of that year, and about 140,000 of those people lived in Edinburgh.

The medieval Old Town endured, and during the 19th Century mouldered into a revolting slum, where 'the windes, down which an English eye may look, but into which no English nose would willingly venture, for stinks older than the Union are to be found there', as Robert Southey wrote in 1819.

Thomas Carlyle, the 'Sage of Ecclefechan', that strange mid-

Victorian thinker and writer, lived for years in that Edinburgh, and knew it well. He wrote that:

> In thrifty Scotland itself, in Glasgow or Edinburgh city, in their dark lanes, hidden from all but the eyes of God, and of rare benevolence by the minister of God, there are scenes of woe, destitution and desolation, such as one may hope, the Sun never saw before in the most barbarous regions where men dwelt.

Of the self-same city, and at about the same time, Alexander Smith wrote:

> Living in Edinburgh there abides, above all things, a sense of its beauty. Hill, crag, castle, rock, blue stretch of sea, the picturesque ridge of the Old Town, the squares and terraces of the New – these things seen once are not to be forgotten. The quick life of today sounding around the relics of antiquity, and overshadowed by the august traditions of a Kingdom, makes residence in Edinburgh more impressive than residence in any other British city. I have just come in – surely it never looked so fair before! What a poem is that Princes Street! The puppets of the busy, many-coloured hour move about on its pavements, while across the ravine Time has piled up the Old Town, ridge on ridge, grey as a rocky coast washed and worn by the foam of centuries; peaked and jagged by gable and roof; windowed from basement to cope, the whole surmounted by St.Giles' airy crown. The New is there looking at the Old. Two Times are brought face to face, and are yet separated by a thousand years. Wonderful on winter nights, when the gully is filled with darkness, and out of it rises, against the sombre blue and the frosty stars, that mass and bulwark of gloom, pierced and quivering with innumerable lights. There is nothing in Europe to match that, I think.

Two writers, two brilliant minds, one city, and two vastly different reports. As Charles Dickens wrote of an earlier century, 'It was the Best of Times; it was the Worst of Times,' and which it was for the individual depended on whether you were born into the grace and beauty or into the misery and ugliness.

Clearly, we are dealing here with virtually two cities: the New Town, with all its grace, beauty and wealth, and the Old Town, shuddering under the weight of hundreds of years of neglect, abject misery and human degradation. It is with the latter we are concerned now, for it was in the Old Town that Duncan Napier worked, set up his shop and his herbal practice, and cured what he could cure, and finally rose out of that human morass to middle class respectability and a moderate wealth.

Central Government – that in London, of course – had reason to fear the city mobs. Riots of various kinds were not uncommon, and it seemed evident that the seeds of revolution could flourish in Great Britain as they had bloomed in France. The Chartist Movement indeed was powerful and represented a threat, it was feared, to good order, although in truth it was mainly a movement of the lower middle classes and skilled artisans. In the early 1840s, the Government ordered reports on the cities, and in 1842, under the editorship of Edwin Chadwick, there appeared *Reports on the Sanitary Conditions of the Labouring Population of Scotland*.

Of Edinburgh, one witness, the very respectable Dr. Alex Miller, stated:

> The dwellings of the poor are generally very filthy... Those of the lowest grade often consist of only one small apartment, always ill-ventilated, both from the nature of its construction and from the densely populated and confined locality in which it is situated. Many of them, besides, are damp and partly underground... A few of the poorest have a bedstead, but by far the larger portion have none; these make up a kind of bed on the floor with straw, on which a whole family are huddled together, some naked and the others in the same clothes they have worn during the day.

One minister of religion, Dr. Lee, testified of Edinburgh that:

> He had never before seen such misery as in his parish, where the people were without furniture, without everything, two married couples often sharing one room. In a single day he had visited seven houses in which there was not a bed, in some of them not

even a heap of straw. Old people of eighty years sleep on the board floor, nearly all slept in their day clothes. In one cellar room, he found two families from a Scotch country district; soon after their removal to the city two of the children had died, and a third was dying at the time of his visit. Each family had a filthy pile of straw lying in a corner; the cellar sheltered besides the two families a donkey, and was moreover so dark that it was impossible to distinguish one person from another by day. Dr. Lee declared that it was enough to make a heart of adamant bleed to see such misery in a country like Scotland.

Those descriptions, of course, are of the poorest of the poor, and it is highly unlikely that many of them were included in the census of 1861. Just a step or two up the economic ladder, the skilled workers and artisans were not really very much better off. That census showed that 34% of all Scottish dwellings had only one room: 37% had two rooms: 1% of families lived in dwellings with no window, and one in five infants born live died before the end of their first year.

A three-volume document was presented to both Houses of Parliament in July 1842. This was a *Report to the Home Secretary from the Poor-Law Commissioners on an Inquiry into the Sanitary Condition of the Labouring Classes in Great Britain*. That wordy title introduced descriptions and figures that were designed to – and did – shock the conscience of mid-Victorian Britain. Of Edinburgh, it said that 'in the dwellings of the poor a want of cleanliness reigns, such as must be expected under those conditions. On the bed-posts chickens roost at night, dogs and horses share the dwellings of human beings, and the natural consequence is a shocking stench, with filth and swarms of vermin.'

The Report went to state that the prevailing construction of Edinburgh favours these atrocious conditions as far as possible:

The Old Town is built upon both slopes of a hill, along the crest of which runs the High Street. Out of the High Street there open downwards multitudes of narrow crooked alleys, called wynds from their many turnings, and these wynds form the proletarian district of the city. The housing of the Scotch [sic] cities, in general, are five or six-storied buildings, like those of Paris, and in contrast with England, where, so far as possible, each family has a separate house. The crowding of human beings upon a limited area is thus intensified.

A contemporary journal reported that:

These streets are often so narrow that a person can step from the window of one house into that of its opposite neighbour, while the houses are piled so high, storey upon storey, that the light can scarcely penetrate to the court or alley that lies between. In this part of the city there are neither sewers nor other drains, nor even privies belonging to the houses. In consequence, all refuse, garbage and excrements of at least 50,000 persons are thrown into the gutters every night, so that, in spite of all street sweeping, a mass of dried filth and foul vapours are created, which not only offend the sight and smell, but endanger the health of the inhabitants in the highest degree. Is it to be wondered at that in such localities all considerations of health, morals and even the most ordinary decency are utterly neglected? On the contrary, all who are more intimately acquainted with the condition of the inhabitants will testify to the high degree which disease, wretchedness and de-moralisation have here reached. Society in such districts has sunk to a level indescribably low and hopeless. The houses of the poor are generally filthy, and are evidently never cleaned. They consist in most cases of a single room which, while subject to the worst ventilation, is yet usually kept cold by the broken and badly fitting windows, and is sometimes damp and partly below ground level, always badly furnished and thoroughly uncomfortable, a straw-heap often serving the whole family for a bed, upon which men and women, young and old, sleep in revolting confusion. Water can be had only from the public pumps, and the difficulty of obtaining it naturally fosters all possible filth.

That report refers to the practice of throwing garbage and

excrement out into the streets below every night. Hence, of course, the infamous Edinburgh cry of 'Gardey Loo!', said to be a corruption of the French *Gardez l'eau*. As a courtesy to those who might be passing below, this was called out of the window before emptying the containers. I have never understood why a corrupted French expression should have been used: there is any number of good Scots phrases that would have sufficed. In any case, wherever possible, the human and animal excrement was stored in a central yard. This was valuable stuff, and local farmers bought it as fertiliser. Their own ordure often paid the rent for those slum dwellers.

However, anyone walking those streets at night certainly had to listen for the dreaded cry, and certainly had to wear special clogs called 'pattens', which had wooden or iron straps lifting the feet a few inches above the accumulated filth.

The misery of those slums was not, of course, confined to Edinburgh. Glasgow, Aberdeen, Dundee and other Scottish cities were in much the same condition. Of Glasgow, it was reported:

> The working class forms here some 78% of the whole population (about 300,000), and lived in parts of the city which exceed in wretchedness and squalor the lowest nooks of St. Giles and Whitechapel, the Liberties of Dublin, the Wynds of Edinburgh. There are numbers of such localities in the heart of the city...endless labyrinths of lanes or wynds into which open at almost every step courts or blind alleys, formed by ill-ventilated, high-piled, waterless and dilapidated houses. These are literally swarming with inhabitants. They contain three or four families upon each floor, perhaps twenty persons. In some cases each storey is let out in sleeping places, so that fifteen to twenty persons are packed, one on top of the other, I cannot say accommodated, in a single room.

A report submitted to the Government by JC Symonds on the condition of hand-loom weavers in Glasgow in 1839 stated:

> I have seen wretchedness in some of its worst phases both here and

upon the Continent, but until I visited the wynds of Glasgow I did not believe that so much crime, misery and disease could exist in any civilised country. In the lower lodging houses, twelve, sometimes twenty persons of both sexes, all ages and various degrees of nakedness, sleep indiscriminately huddled together upon the floor. These dwellings are usually so damp, filthy and ruinous, that no one could wish to keep his horse in one of them...

The wynds of Glasgow contain a fluctuating population of fifteen to thirty thousand human beings. This quarter consists wholly of narrow alleys and square courts, in the middle of every one of which lies a dung heap. Revolting as was the outward appearance of those courts, I was yet not prepared for the filth and wretchedness within. In some of the sleeping-places which we visited at night....we found a complete layer of human beings stretched upon the floor, often fifteen to twenty, some clad, others naked, men and women indiscriminately. Their bed was a litter of mouldy straw, mixed with rags.

There was little or no furniture, and the only thing which gave these dens any shimmer of habitableness was a fire upon the hearth. Theft and prostitution form the chief means of subsistence of this population. No one seems to take the trouble to cleanse this Augean stable, this Pandemonium, this tangle of crime, filth and pestilence, in the centre of the second city of the kingdom.

Naturally, these deplorable living conditions led to ill-health and death. Good health and longevity are the products of many things, and certainly reasonable housing and clothing, adequate food, clean water and the availability of medical assistance are amongst them. Those Wretched of the Earth in the city slums had none of these. Their housing we have described; their clothing we can imagine; their food we would reject with horror – half-rotten potatoes, stinking fish, adulterated milk laden with bacteria, mouldy bread made from flour mixed with chalk

The appalling cholera and typhus epidemics of the 1830s and 1840s had ended, but the mortality rates were still very high. Children under ten years of age accounted for 54% of all deaths in 1861. Tuberculosis was still rampant, and was the major cause of death. Respiratory diseases of various kinds were close behind. As already noted, the records of the Edinburgh Royal Infirmary show that many patients were admitted suffering only from neglect and malnutrition, and they were kept in hospital long enough to be cleaned up and reasonably well fed, before being returned to their old conditions. Incidentally, as a small matter of interest, one of the treatments used in the Royal Infirmary in those days was acupuncture.

Inevitably, in the deplorable conditions in which those people lived, many turned to drink as a brief escape from reality. Those aged fifteen and over drank, on average, about a pint (500ml) of whisky each week. Since many women did not drink, and nor did a minority of men, those who did drink must have had a considerable consumption. And that, of course, was duty-paid whisky: there is no way of estimating the consumption of illegally produced spirits. In those days, methylated spirit was not the highly coloured and vomit-inducing liquid we know today, and it was the basis for home-production, by pub and club managers, of much 'whisky'. Meths, sugar, water and the Essence of Prune (a popular laxative of the day) was the formula for that liquor. Heaven knows what that infernal brew did to the constitution of those who drank it regularly, but, as one observer noted, 'It offers a transient escape from the miseries of life and brings the only moments of comparative happiness which they ever enjoy.' In Old Testament days, Lemuel's mother offered advice to her son: 'Let him drink and forget his poverty, and remember his misery no more.'

That wonderful writer on Scotland, Neil Gunn, had a perceptive comment on excessive drinking:

> One wonders why those who were (and still are) repelled abhorrently by whisky were not infinitely more repelled by the social conditions which let whisky act so revealingly. One would think that whisky had been the cause of the state of the poor, that it had built the slums and ensured the poverty, that it was the whole monstrous creator of that economic hell... One may readily have patience with the women, who, being realists, condemned the drunken horrors they saw. But with the so-called

social and temperance reformers, as with the religious and political rulers, patience is less easy, for it is natural to expect that they would have made some effort to see through the effect to the causes, and, once having seen, to have become the people's impassioned leaders against the savagery of a system that produced such appalling results.

But not only did they support the social order (many seeing in it the righteous handiwork of a God who had called each to his appointed place), but were themselves of the owning or governing class who hunted and persecuted such 'friends of the people' as, haunted by humanity's vision of liberty and fraternity, dared raise a voice in the peoples' favour.

That might well have been so, but there can be little doubt that drinking to excess produced a great deal of domestic violence, prostitution, theft and other crime.

To sum up, Edinburgh, that beautiful city of gracious squares and crescents, of lovely vistas and hills, that Athens of the North, also contained human degradation and incredible poverty of a nature and intensity we can hardly comprehend today. It was virtually into the middle of those stews and hovels that Duncan Napier stepped in 1860, with his herbs and his little shop, and with his incredible courage to walk the few hundred yards down into the Grassmarket on Saturday nights and preach the virtues of temperance to the drunken, fighting, vomiting crowds.

PART III

Napiers of Edinburgh

Widow Welch's Pills

A sovereign remedy for all female complaints, nervous disorders, weakness of the solids, loss of appetite, sick headache, lowness of spirits and particularly for irregularities in the female system.

Part of a poster and handbill widely distributed in mid-Victorian Edinburgh.

WIDOW WELCH'S PILLS, Morrison's Pills, Dr. Mainwaring's Pills, Parr's Life Pills – the whole of mid-Victorian Britain was flooded with 'patent medicines'. We really cannot know now what most of those concoctions contained, although certainly sugar and chalk were much used. Some were probably inert and harmless, others not. There were many laxatives, of course, and others for 'Period Pains Peculiar to Women'. Many others, like Widow Welch's, were for 'irregularities in the female system', a coded message that they just might bring on a delayed menstruation, or, in other words, deal with a suspected and unwanted pregnancy.

Whoever thought up the name for 'Parr's Life Pills' was something of an early advertising genius. The name obviously links the pills with the famous Thomas 'Old' Parr, who allegedly lived to the age of 152. He married his second wife when he was 120, worked every day until he was 130, and eventually was taken to London to the court of Charles I, and there treated so royally that he died of it. Take Parr's Life Pills, then, and live as long as Old Parr himself! Just why anyone would want to live so long in the pullulating misery amongst which the customers existed is not obvious. Still, many people must have done, for 20-25,000 boxes were sold each week.

Some of those patent medicines were not so innocuous. The

active ingredient of Godfrey's Cordial, for example, was laudanum, and it was used chiefly to soothe children. Laudanum, of course, is an extract of opium, and certainly would keep children quiet and well-soothed. It would also cause them to become addicted. One apothecary alone is reported to have used 13 cwt (660 kilograms) of laudanum each year in preparing that cordial alone.

According to its label in 1876, Mrs. Lydia E Pinkham's Pills for Pale People was 'vegetable compound for Prolapsus Uteri, or Falling of the Womb, and all Female Weaknesses, including Leucorrhea (Vaginal Discharge), Painful Menstruation, Inflammation and Ulceration of the Womb, Irregularities, Flooding, and Etc.'

Oddly enough, almost a hundred years later, Mrs. Lydia E Pinkham's Pills for Pale People were recalled in a popular song of the 1960s. It was, I think, a group called The Scaffold who sang:

We'll drink a drink a drink
To Lily the Pink the Pink the Pink
The saviour of the human race
For she invented a medicinal compound
Most efficacious in every case.

Not only were the corner shops full of those dubious concoctions, but the travelling medicine men were to be seen in every market and in the crowded Saturday night streets. Usually well-dressed and laden with 'gold' bracelets, necklaces and rings, or exotically garbed as Red Indians or African chiefs, they offered magic relief from all pains and aches: 'It's good for what ails you, and if nothing ails you, it's good for that, too!' Only one drop of the amazing Jamborozo Tincture would instantly stop a toothache, a teaspoonful would ease the rheumatics, one bottle would end the uncertainty worrying the young woman. And there was always someone in the crowd willing to be treated there and then, after listening to the entertaining patter of the 'Professor' or 'Doctor' or even 'Prince'. And then the shillings and the bottles changed hands and the poor and sick had hope for another week. And then the Prince and his 'patient' went off together to recuperate in the dram-shop. Those entertaining and probably harm-less characters continued to visit the street markets of Britain until the World War of 1939.

Of course, for those really ill, there was always the hospital, but the hospital was a place to be feared. The treatments offered could be extreme, perhaps worse than the illness. Almost certainly you would be bled until syncope threatened – a fainting fit or even incipient heart failure. You might be lucky, and have someone try out the new Galvanism on you – an electric shock which caused involuntary movements of the limbs. If you had a wound, or had suffered the agony of an amputation, then probably cauterisation would be used to seal the blood vessels – the application of a white hot iron. Those perhaps a little luckier would instead have a 'Potential Cauterisation', that is, the application to the wound of a very caustic liquid. Cataplasms, which the lay person called 'poultices', were much used, and were applied, and kept, very hot. Perhaps the doctor would prescribe a good blistering to relieve chronic pain, and for this cantharides, the highly irritating Spanish Fly, was popular. A turpentine enema must have been compara-tively gentle, and the application of leeches to a shaven head prob-ably welcome as a relief. The really lucky would be treated with acupuncture, but those with little hope would receive regular pre-scriptions of red wine or spirits.

It is not surprising that Napoleon is said to have told his Chief Physician that Medicine, in those days, was the science of mur-derers.

For those rich enough, there was no shortage of professional medical help in mid-Victorian Edinburgh, and for the poor there was a plethora of self-help medication. Each was probably as effective as the other.

It was into this field of sickness that Duncan Napier decided to enter in 1860, at the age of 29. A baker by trade, he had suf-fered much ill-treatment at the hands of his adoptive mother dur-ing his childhood and as a youth. He had early developed an inter-est in gardening, and from that a great interest in botany and in the use of herbs for healing. He read widely, and was soon an enthusiastic and prominent member of the Edinburgh Botanical

Society. He began treating himself and his family with the herbs he gathered around Edinburgh, and then others, like his workmates, began to seek his help and advice in treating their illnesses. Soon, he was treating so many, and so successfully and cheaply, that he decided to take the chance of opening a herb shop and setting up as a herbalist.

Prudently, he kept on with his day job, and worked in his shop only in the evenings, with his wife serving there during the day. He spent whatever spare hours he had in tramping the hills around the city, gathering the herbs he used in his treatments. As a journeyman baker, and newly married, he had no capital and no savings, and it was really not surprising that he found it impossible to get any financial assistance until he approached his friend John Hope.

That philanthropic man loaned Duncan enough money to pay rent on his shop, and also to stock it and provide a financial cushion until it was successful – or failed. But it did not fail. Instead, it flourished, and soon Duncan had enough self-confidence to give up the baking trade and work full-time at his chosen profession of herbalist.

The shop Duncan chose was in Bristo Place, Edinburgh. The unusual name is probably derived from the 'brewsters' who originally had settled there. It was an area then verging on some of the worst slums, and yet already showing some signs of regeneration. The city Bedlam – Lunatic Asylum – was there, and the poet Robert Fergusson died in that hell-hole. Robert Burns knew Bristo Place well, for not only did he arrange and pay for a headstone over the grave of his fellow-poet Robert Fergusson in the nearby Greyfriars Kirkyard, but he made many clandestine visits to Mrs. Agnes McLehose who lodged there, and was the 'Clarinda' of that strange and hectic correspondence between Clarinda and Sylvander, Burns, of course, being Sylvander. In one letter Clarinda warns Sylvander against visiting her at night, the area being unsafe.

That first shop was not the present premises of Napiers. After fourteen years of a growing practice, and a growing demand for his herbs, it was necessary to have much bigger premises, and Duncan moved along the street to the corner in 1874. That second shop is still the headquarters and indeed the flagship of Napiers of Edinburgh.

Above the doorway of the shop a stone plaque still notes that, in 1513, it was the site of the Town Wall, that is, the Flodden Wall, built belatedly to protect the city from English incursions after the disastrous defeat of Flodden Field in 1513. Highlanders and Lowlanders, led by James IV, fought together that day, and went down to total defeat by Henry VIII's army.

There were already herbalists practising in Edinburgh when Duncan opened his shop. Four other herbal shops and practices have been traced, and those appear to have been Thomsonian or Coffinite. None of them was very successful. The outlook for Duncan was hardly bright, and he was well advised to keep his day job as a baker while he sought to establish himself as a professional healer.

Duncan was a wonderful example of an autodidact. With very little formal education, he became an acknowledged expert in his chosen field of herbal healing. More than that, though, he developed very strong views on religion and morality, and was never afraid to express them in public. Much later, he wrote an autobiography which was never completed or published (see Appendix IV). His handwriting was clear, firm and legible, although not the lovely copper-plate that the teachers of the day – and long afterwards – insisted on. He was prepared to go prison for his beliefs.

To quote from an obituary of Duncan published in *Potter's Bulletin* in April 1921:

> By nature a fighter, he was a man of strong conviction; one of the foremost in opposing the vaccination compulsory laws for non-compliance with which he was fined several times; a staunch Protestant, a stout Free Churchman; an ardent opponent of the laws of the Church of Rome, taking the chair at most of the Anti-Popery meetings in the city.

In his early days as a healer, he appears to have been strongly influenced by the teachings of both Samuel Thomson and Albert Coffin, and seems to have reconciled the principles of both.

Did he apply the steamings which were an integral part of Thomsonianism? That could not have been easy in the crowded Edinburgh tenements. Surely, though, when he took the decision to open his shop and clinic, he would have echoed the words of Samuel Thomson: 'I finally concluded to make use of that gift which I thought the God of Nature had implanted in me.'

Samuel Thomson's favourite herb was lobelia, which he used as an emetic, after a course of sweating and treatment with other herbs. He argued that his treatments, by restoring the animal warmth of the body, had thrown the sickness to the stomach, from which it was removed by the vomiting produced by the lobelia. Perhaps today we raise a cynical eyebrow at the theory: we cannot be cynical about the undoubted results of his treatments.

It is interesting that Duncan cured his first patient – himself – with lobelia, Samuel Thomson's favourite herb. He had been troubled with a persistent cough since his boyhood, and, reading about Lobelia Syrup as a cough cure in his precious *Brooke's Family Herbal* (published as a part-book at two pence per copy), he tried to buy the herb from an Edinburgh chemist. They refused to supply it, on the grounds that it was a poison, so Duncan obtained it from Dr. Albert Coffin's Herbal Warehouse in London. He prepared his first Lobelia Syrup in a seven-pound sweetie jar.

The syrup certainly cured his cough, although the cure was hardly painless, since he vomited every morning. However, perseverance paid, and after six months he was cured, proving wrong his auld wifie neighbours who had said that the poor laddie could not live long with such a graveyard cough. Eighty years later he was still hale and hearty, and still prescribing his Lobelia Cough Syrup, and incidentally selling it in wholesale quantities to the Edinburgh chemists who had refused to supply him with his first two ounces of lobelia herb.

Circumstantially, then, it seems safe to assume that Duncan knew of, and learned from the teachings of both Samuel Thomson and Albert Coffin, and that he also drew what he thought best from his other reading. Indeed, how else could he have learned his trade? There were no schools of Herbal Medicine then, and no Universities offering degrees in the art. Even if formal training as a herbalist had been available, there was no way Duncan could have utilised it. He was a young married man with a family, and a baker to trade. His hours of work were long and no doubt arduous. He had little money. He had herbs to collect and dry in their due season. He had some patients to visit. He had his books to study. There could hardly have been enough hours in each day for him, nor enough days in the week. The Sabbath, of course, was not for work or study of his herbal books.

In his own writings, Duncan gave little indication of the books he studied. However, a few remnants of his library remain, and they indicate a wide range of interests. There is a pamphlet, *A Note on Jaborandi: A Paper* read by William Craig M.D. Etc., Lecturer on Materia Medica at the Edinburgh School of Medicine, at the Medico-Chirugical Society of Edinburgh on 10th November 1875. (Jaborandi was a newly imported Brazilian herb, which, Dr Craig found, had 'remarkable powers as a sialogogue and diaphoretic.' That is, it increases the production of saliva and promotes sweating. In spite of Dr Craig's enthusiasm for it, the herb was never widely used, perhaps because of problems in procuring the pure, unadulterated herb. It is not used today in Western herbalism, except as an occasional treatment for glaucoma.)

Another pamphlet is *Remarks on the Mustard Tree of Scripture, a Paper* read before the Asiatic Society. The author, R Brown Esq, presented the copy to Duncan 'With the Writer's Respects' in the 1860s.

A booklet, *The Indigenous Drugs of India* by Kanny Lol Dey, Teacher at the Medical College of Calcutta, was printed by Thacker, Spink and Co, Calcutta, in 1867.

There is a *List of Medicinal and Poisonous Plants Cultivated in the Royal Botanic Garden of Edinburgh, 1859.*

There is a reprinted extract from the Pharmaceutical Journal of May 1877, '*The Medicinal Plants of Scotland*', by the same Dr. Craig who introduced Jaborandi.

Another extract from the *Pharmaceutical Journal*, for October 1889 is '*Botanical and Pharmacological Inquiries and Desiderata*', by Sir William J Hooker, Director of the Royal Gardens of Kew.

Although Duncan's Bristo Place shop was at first open only in the evenings, it very soon became clear that the demand for his herbs and his healing skills was considerable and growing. So, with some trepidation, he decided to give up the baking trade, and open the shop full time. Wisely, though, he arranged with his employer that if the business failed, he could go back to the baking trade.

His precautions, and perhaps also his doubts, were unnecessary. The shop and his practice as a herbalist flourished, and very soon customers and patients were queuing for his services. Although now freed from the servitude of the baking trade, his hours of work were still very long, sometimes impossibly so. As the business and practice grew, so of course did the demand for herbs, and most of those were still collected by Duncan himself.

As Duncan's practice grew, so, clearly, did his knowledge, and in 1868 that self-taught man achieved Registration as a Chemist and Druggist, and a year later he was elected a Member of the Medical Reformers of England.

Duncan's eldest son, Andrew Nelson Napier, joined his father in the business in 1870, and continued to practice as a highly trained professional herbalist for the next 50 years. It was Andrew's son Charles who painted a portrait of Duncan as a patriarchal old man, and that portrait became, and remains, the symbol of Napiers.

Charles, a Member of the Royal Society of Watercolorists, produced a work of art that is truly memorable. It depicts a leonine, heavily-bearded man of somewhat ruddy complexion. But it is the eyes which are most impressive. Piercing yet still gentle and kindly, they seem to indicate sympathy and understanding. Certainly it is the head of a man who could be trusted to help and heal.

It is also the head of a man who endured much and suffered much. Not only was he brought up, if that is the right expression, by uncaring and sadistic adoptive parents, but two of his children died, apparently as a result of being vaccinated against smallpox. A law compelling the vaccination of all children was enacted in 1853, and after the death of his two sons, Duncan steadfastly refused, as he wrote, 'to have any more of my children vaccinated, and run the terrible risk of this death, or ill-health, as a material consequence, for to my certain knowledge some hundreds of children have been killed though this vile operation.' He was quite prepared to go to jail, or be fined, for his convictions.

Duncan's autobiography apparently contained an account of those deaths, but some unknown hand has removed the pages, leaving only a bare description of the death of his first son, John, and very shortly afterwards the death of the younger son, Duncan. Two daughters also caught smallpox, but both survived.

Of course, Duncan was by no means alone in his battle against vaccination. Virtually all the alternative practitioners in the country united in the Anti-Vaccination League, and they were joined by many regular doctors. It was a battle conducted with a vehemence and a degree of vituperation unknown to us today. The editor of one provincial newspaper wrote an article critical of the Anti-Vaccination League. The next issue of the *British Medical Reform Association Journal* attacked him as 'a weak-minded scribbler', an 'abettor of the vast tribe of Blood Poisoners,' 'a pettifogging scribe', an 'imbecile Editor', a 'foggy-minded Editor', and a 'vociferous and contemptible creature'. We should not be surprised at such vehemence, since the anti-vaccinationists were thoroughly convinced, with some reason, that vaccination, as then practised, was a highly dangerous, perhaps deadly, operation.

The problem lay with the lymph, the vaccine, which was extracted at first from cows infected with cowpox, and then from infected humans. It needed to be carefully stored, kept cold, and used fresh, and very often it wasn't. Such careful treatment must have been difficult in those days even for hospitals and trained doctors: the ministers and their wives, and the lairds' wives who seemed to view vaccination of their flocks as a hobby or a duty certainly could not have stored or treated the lymph as it required.

The lymph from infected humans could also carry with it the infection of syphilis, and there could be no doubt that, as Duncan so stoutly proclaimed, such vaccination was no more than the introduction of blood poisoning to an otherwise healthy body. Duncan records several deaths which he believed to be due to vaccination, and wrote that he knew of hundreds more, and he was only one practitioner in only one city. Even the proponents of vaccination, in their official reports, admitted there were problems.

Vaccination, they wrote, causes a mild fever and a constitutional disturbance in all cases, reaching a height about the eighth day. General vaccinia, it was noted, occurs in about one in every 30,000 subjects, and post-vaccinal encephalitis in one in every 50,000, and admitted that both are serious complications.

It was hardly surprising that Duncan and his fellow members of the Anti-Vaccination League struggled against it.

Although he seems to have never taken an active part in the organisation, Duncan remained a full member of what was by then the British Medical Reform Association, which proclaimed 'The New Era of Eclecticism'. The list of members shows only Duncan and two other members in Scotland, one also in Edinburgh, and the other in Dundee.

The Eclectics, as the name implies, did not adhere to any single theory of botanical healing, but chose from each what they considered appropriate in each case. Coffinites, Thomsonians, Beachites, and those who used only the simple remedies of ancient tradition were united for the first time, in one organisation, and could speak with one voice in defence of their beliefs and their profession.

We know little of Duncan's views on subjects other than herbalism, teetotalism and religion. However, it is surely significant that his sons all displayed a deep Scottish patriotism, and it is reasonable to suppose that they imbibed this at home. This patriotism did not evince itself as nationalism in any form, but rather as the sort of deep love of their country and its traditions shown by Sir Walter Scott in his writing. It was a romantic view of the country and its history, with emphasis on the pageantry and colour, the Highland dress, the wearing of the kilt and all the other external symbols of Scottishness.

There is only one small indicator of Duncan's political views. Amongst his papers is a booklet, well-thumbed and repaired. It is headed 'PRIVATE: For Use of Members Only', and was published in November 1897 by the Traders' Defence Association of Scotland. It declares itself to be '*The Third List of Manufacturers and Wholesale Merchants who are acting on the principle of Non-Employment of co-operative Labour.*' The Board of Management addressed the Members:

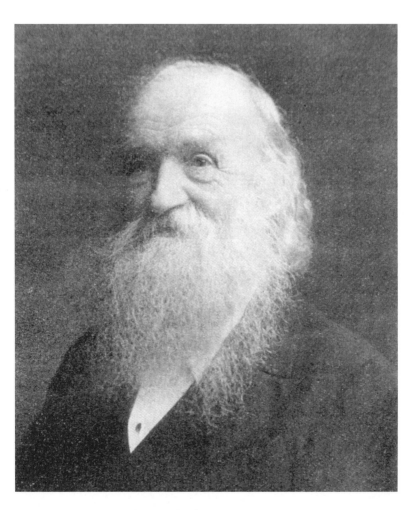

Duncan Napier, 1831 to 1921

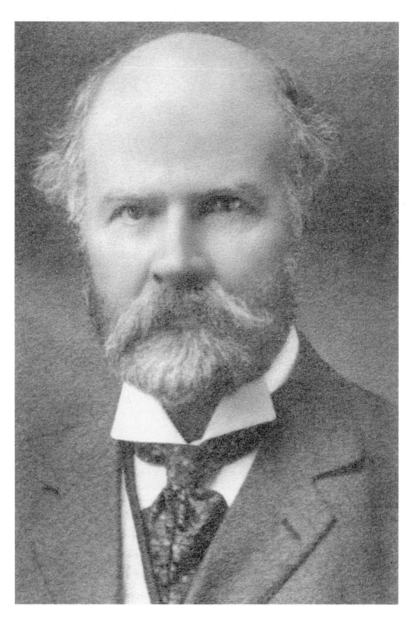

Andrew Nelson Napier, 1867 to 1916

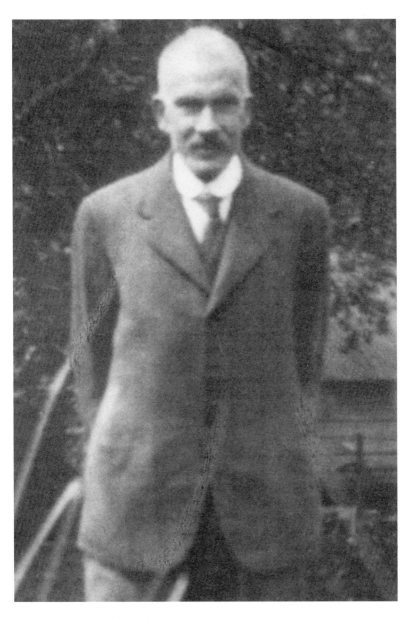

Walter Glendinning Napier, 1872 to 1934

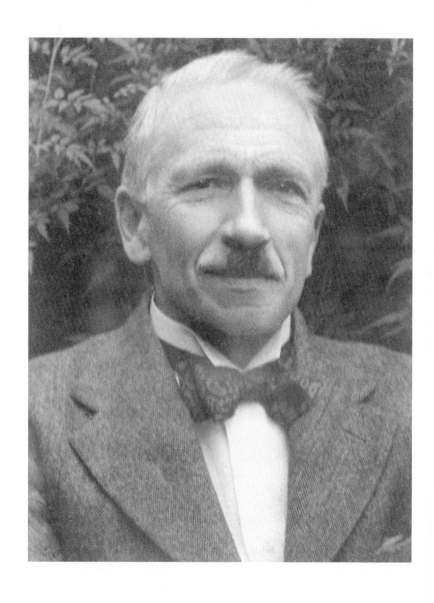

Duncan Scott Napier, 1900 to 1956

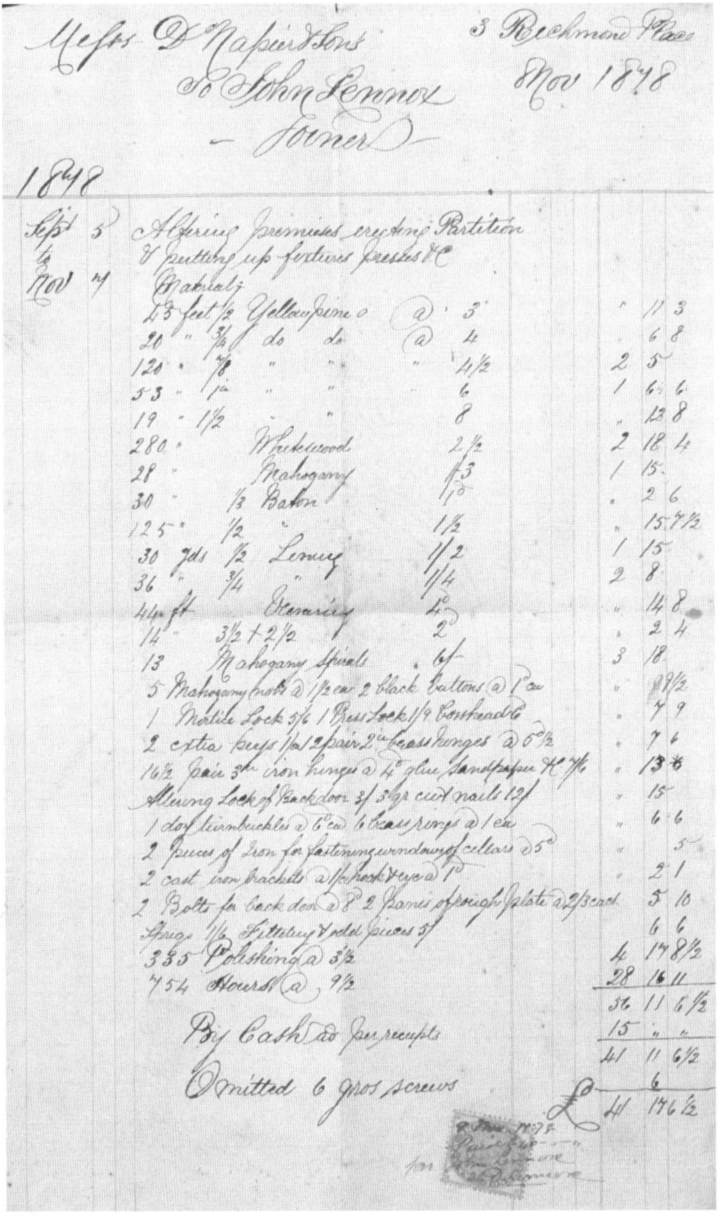

Messrs D Napier & Sons 3 Richmond Place
To John Lennox 8 Nov 1878
— Joiner —

1878

Sept 5 to Nov 4 Altering premises erecting Partition & putting up fixtures presses &c
Materials

		£	s	d
45 feet 1/2 Yellow pine	@ 3	"	11	3
20 " 3/4 do do	@ 4	"	6	8
120 " 7/8 " "	4 1/2	2	5	
53 " 1 " "	6	1	6	6
19 " 1 1/2 "	8	"	12	8
280 " Whitewood	2 1/2	2	18	4
28 " Mahogany	1/3	1	15	
30 " 1/3 Baton	1d	"	2	6
125 " 1/2 "	1 1/2	"	15	7 1/2
30 yds 1/2 Lenning	1/2	1	15	
36 " 3/4 "	1/4	2	8	
44 ft Ovaries	4d	"	14	8
14 " 3 1/2 + 2 1/2	2d	"	2	4
13 Mahogany Spirals	6/	3	18	
5 Mahogany knobs @ 1/2 ea 2 black buttons @ 1d ea		"		8 1/2
1 Mortise Lock 5/6 1 Press Lock 1/9 Countersunk		"	7	9
2 extra keys 1/- 12 pair 2in brass hinges @ 6d 1/2		"	7	6
16 1/2 pair 3in iron hinges @ 4d glue sandpaper &c 7/6		"	13	6
Altering Lock of back door 3/ 3 lb cut nails 12/		"	15	
1 doz turnbuckles @ 6d ea 6 brass rings @ 1 ea		"	6	6
2 pieces of Iron for fastening windows of cellars @ 5d		"		5
2 cast iron brackets @ 1/- hook & eye @ 1d		"	2	1
2 Bolts for back door @ 8d 2 panes of rough plate @ 2/3 each			5	10
Sprigs 1/6 Fitting & odd pieces 5/			6	6
335 Polishing @ 3 1/2		4	17	8 1/2
754 Hours @ 9 1/2		28	16	11
		56	11	6 1/2
By Cash as per receipts		15	"	"
		41	11	6 1/2
Omitted 6 gros screws			6	
	£	41	17	6 1/2

Account for renovation of clinic and shop in 1878

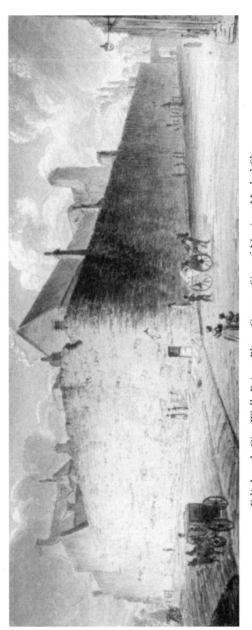

Edinburgh City Wall, Bristo Place Corner. Site of Napiers Herbal Shop.

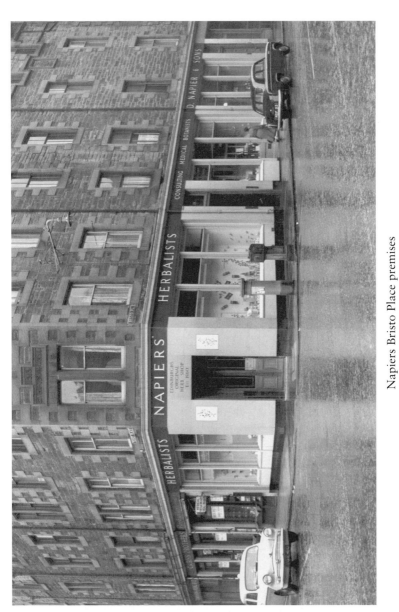

Napiers Bristo Place premises

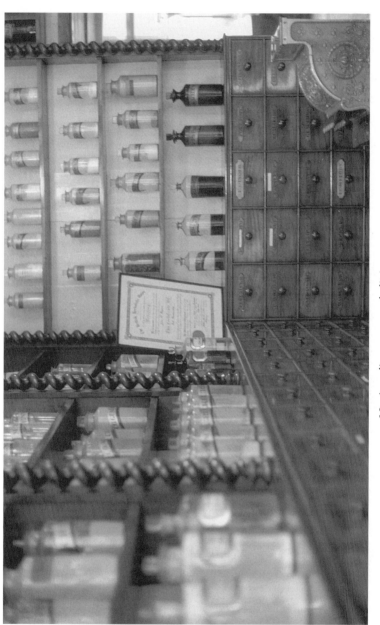

Napiers dispensary and clinic

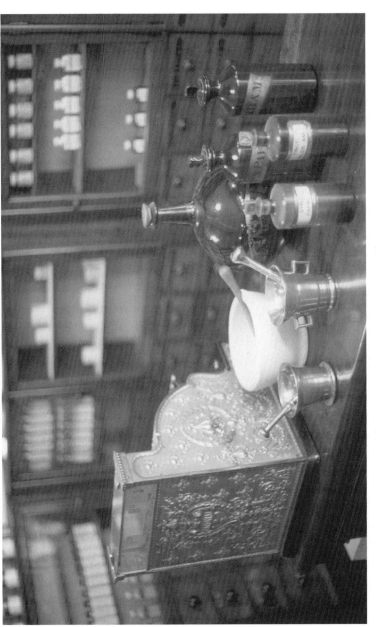

The Dispensary, Napiers, 18 Bristo Place. 1960

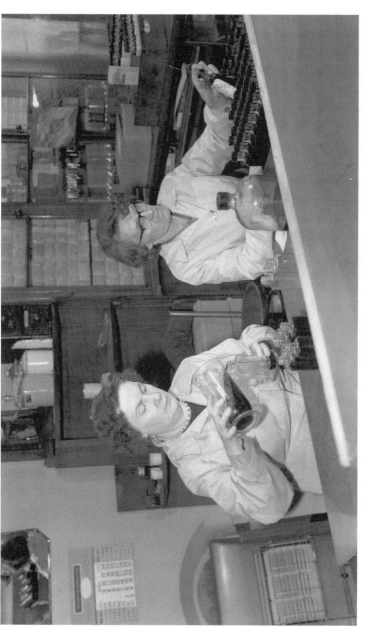

Lobelia Cough Syrup being bottled and packed for wholesale distribution. c1960

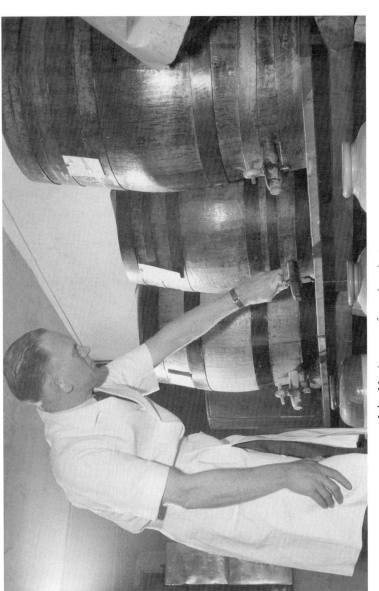

John Napier manufacturing tinctures. c1970

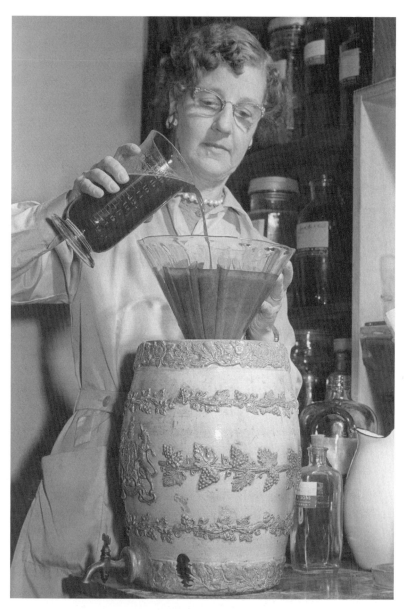

Filtering No2 Hair Lotion. c1970
This product is still one of Napiers best sellers.

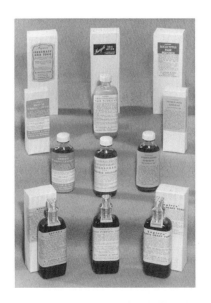

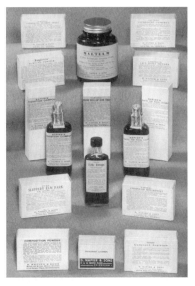

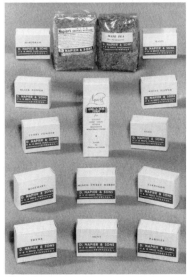

Napiers Mail Order Catalogue pages. c1950

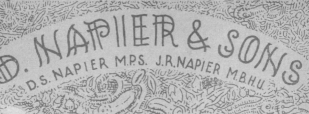

Handbill advertising Napiers. c1930

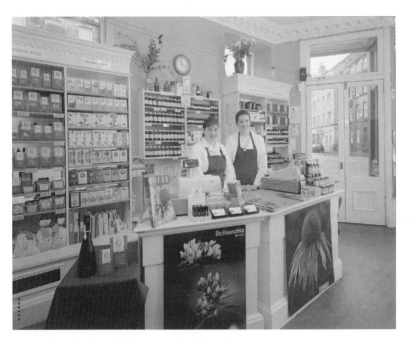

Napiers, Hamilton Place, 2003

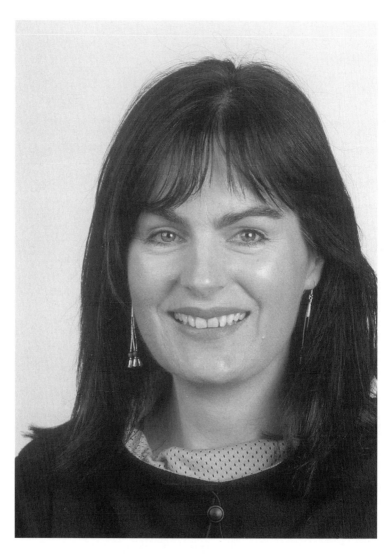

Dee Atkinson

[We] urge you as strongly as words can, to deal only with those whose names are here enrolled, and pay no heed to those who hypocritically express sympathy with our work and endeavour to explain away the absence from the List of the name of the Firms they represent, their purpose being to secure business from the private trader while they are sedulously cultivating the trade of the Co-operative Stores.

The list of members of this rather peculiar body does not include the firm of Duncan Napier, nor indeed any other herbalist, although it does include many trades, from Aerated Water Manufacturers to Yarn Factors, from Potted Head Makers to Coffee Essence Producers. The members are asked to use only the Caledonian and London North Western Railways for carriage of their goods, and to travel on those lines when possible. It gives no indication of why those two particular railways were favoured, but we may suppose that the other railways committed the offence of carrying the goods of the rapidly growing Co-operative movement.

If we can only infer Duncan's political views on very slender evidence, there can be no doubts about his views on drinking. From his youth to his death he was a vehement advocate of teetotalism.

Considering his up-bringing, this is hardly surprising. He saw at first hand the effects of excessive drinking, and suffered many a flogging from a drunkard adoptive mother. Living in a drinking den, he was surrounded by drink, and by his own account drank nothing but beer until his early youth.

It was his relationship with John Hope that changed his course, not only to a total abstention from alcohol and tobacco but also to a rigid Protestant Christianity. It was during Duncan's early morning deliveries of fresh rolls that he frequently met and talked with John Hope. Those early morning meetings were also indirectly responsible for the establishment of Napiers Herbalists, for without the financial support of that philanthropic man, Duncan might very well have found it impossible to open his first shop.

There is no doubt that by the beginning of the 19th century, drink permeated Scotland at all levels. From the highest to the lowest elements of society, from the Highlands to the Central Belt and on to the Lowlands, every activity and event seemed to require lubrication with copious amounts of alcohol. Judges carried their bottles of claret with them to the bench: ministers freed their thoughts and their tongues with a good dram before entering the pulpit, and were esteemed for their ability to hold their liquor. As the ancient joke has it, when the old stalwart of the kirk visited the new minister for the first time, he reported back to his cronies: 'Ah, he's a grand man! He opened a new bottle and he threw the cork into the fire!' Births, marriages and deaths were the occasions for drinking, and so were starting new jobs or ending old ones.

However, it was not the social drinking of the middle and upper classes that kindled the flames of the temperance movement, and nor was it the occasional drinking that marked important events in life and death. Such drinking was sedate enough, and usually in secret. It was the public and excessive drinking of the poor, the slum dwellers, that caused concern.

There was certainly good reason for that concern. There are many contemporary accounts of the regular drunken debauchery in the slum areas of mid-Victorian Scotland, and although they are almost without exception written by the advocates of temperance or teetotalism, and thus perhaps biased, they do present a picture of alcoholic excess difficult to understand today. Nor can there by any doubt that the compulsion to drink led to much theft and prostitution – much like the picture today of those addicted to other drugs.

The temperance movement began as just that – a plea for temperance in drinking, not its prohibition. The movement rapidly became less tolerant, and soon all alcohol, beer, spirits and wine, became the Demon Drink. The movement for total abstinence once embraced tens of thousands of men, women and children.

In 1842, Father Theobald Mathew, the 'Irish Apostle of Temperance' as he was known, visited Glasgow. It was estimated that 50,000 people travelled by rail from all over the Central Belt to hear him preach on Glasgow Green, and as a result, in three days 40,000 people signed the pledge to abstain from alcohol, and many of them were Irish Catholics, like Father Mathew himself.

This was particularly interesting, since it was widely believed that Irish immigrants were the hardest and most obstreperous drinkers. The census of 1841 had listed 125,000 Irish-born inhabitants of Scotland, and that was almost certainly an underestimate. A little later the Irish famine drove up to 1,000 more each week into Glasgow. Mostly unskilled, they could occupy only the lowest levels of labour in the booming mills and factories. Living in the worst of the housing, they came to have a reputation for fighting, drunkenness and 'general bad behaviour'.

Furthermore, since they were unorganised and desperate, they were regarded as a vital source of cheap labour, and were often used as strike breakers. In 1846 the Scottish iron workers had been on strike for fourteen long weeks, resisting a cut in wages. Irish immigrants took their place, the strike was broken, and wages in the iron mills reduced from five shillings to three shillings a day. This reinforced the view that the Irish were a threat to Scottish well-being, and it was a short and simple step from that to the development of a sectarianism that still bedevils the nation.

There was an occasional voice raised to protest that the temperance movement had got it wrong, that drink was not the cause of the degradation of the slum dwellers, but rather that the slum conditions led inevitably to the temporary escape of drinking. They were solitary voices in a vast desert of misunderstanding, though, and efforts to alleviate the undoubted problem were always directed to controlling it, and not to abolish the cause. Besides, of course, it was much cheaper and easier to turn the drinking dens into unpleasant places where men congregated to get drunk, than to tackle the enormous problem of the slum housing. That had to wait for another hundred years.

Duncan, with the courage of a zealot, had no hesitation in preaching his gospel of total abstinence. He had the practise of closing his shop at ten o'clock on Saturday evenings, walking the few hundred yards to Edinburgh's Grassmarket, and there, in the midst of drunkenness and debauchery, attempting to make converts, and save the bodies and souls of his audience.

We do not know whether he made converts. We cannot tell whether any who came to scoff left convinced. One thing, though, is certain: it took considerable courage to do what he did. Perhaps only his growing reputation as a healer, and one who never turned away a penniless patient, saved him from the brickbats and flung horse dung which other vocal teetotallers endured. On more than one occasion, though, he was extricated by the police from jeering crowds.

Although the reason for Duncan's campaign against the Demon Drink can be easily understood, his very public campaign against the Roman Catholic Church remains puzzling. Again, John Hope seems to have been responsible for Duncan's acceptance of a rather strict form of Protestantism, but John Hope does not figure in the Anti-Popery campaigns into which Duncan plunged with enthusiasm – such enthusiasm indeed that he became a prominent speaker and leader of those campaigns.

Certainly the purity of Scottish Calvinism was being much diluted by Catholic, mainly Irish, immigration into the industrial areas of Scotland. It is easy to understand why the working class and working class organisations such as Trade Unions saw the Catholics as a threat. It is not so easy to understand why the middle classes (and Duncan by now was well established as middle class) were often so vehement about the 'Roman Threat'.

Of course, Scotland had long been polarised by religious divisions, and much blood had been shed in religious struggles. That polarisation increased dramatically as a result of Victorian Catholic immigration, and this seemed to lead to a revival of old memories of many wicked deeds. Whatever the reasons, and some of them seem to lie deep in the Scottish psyche, Anti-Popery and Anti-Catholic feelings ran strong in those years. They still do, to some extent. Duncan, with characteristic courage, voiced them publicly. After all, it was only a few years earlier that the plaque marking the site where the Great Fire of London started, attributed that fire to 'the treachery and malice of the popish faction.'

So the Bristo Place shop was successful. Duncan and his family lived comfortably in Ruby Villa, Sciennes, a well-to-do suburb. There was a large garden at Ruby Villa, and Duncan was able to revert to his first love, growing things, especially herbs used in the practice. This did not mean that the gathering of herbs from the wild ended. As the practice grew, so did the herb-gathering expeditions, and the whole family was involved in it. Wherever they went in Scotland – and they travelled far – herbs were gathered and transformed into medicines.

The eldest surviving son, Andrew Nelson Napier, entered the business in 1870, and served as a herbalist until his death in 1916. A photograph of him shows a moustached and bearded man, balding, and dressed in the conventional stiff wing collar and neatly knotted tie of the professional man of the period. Unlike those of his father Duncan, Andrew's eyes are sharp and piercing. He was said to have been a loveable and genial character with a great love of his garden, whose hobby was collecting china and pictures. He was well-known in Edinburgh as a patron of art and music.

Duncan's youngest son, also Duncan Scott Napier, was born in 1879, educated at George Watson's College, and then qualified as a chemist before entering the business. The three men, Duncan, Andrew Scott and Duncan II entered into a formal partnership in 1905. Duncan Napier, Herbalist became DS Napier & Sons, Herbalists.

An elder son, Walter Glendinning Napier, born in 1872, was also educated at George Watson's College, and then graduated MA and BSC from the University of Edinburgh with honours in Natural Philosophy and Botany. Walter, who proved to be a brilliant tutor, seemed destined for an academic career, but it was not to be.

Long afterwards, in 1946, Duncan II had a book privately printed. This book, *Memorable Days*, reads perhaps rather strangely today, with its emphasis on *mens sano in corpore sano* – a healthy mind in a healthy body – and its openly declared version of Muscular Christianity. In the book, Walter, or Big, as he seems to have been known, is described as:

> A big, upstanding lad he was, half an inch under six feet in his stockings, a forty-two inch chest, lean in the flank and a sixteen inch calf. Inclined to be stiff in his flat back he had a tremendous reach, as I knew so well when fencing with him, and there were few could tire him at the walking.

> I was just the average uninteresting boy, sensitive and high strung, mad on gymnastics and being a strong man. We wore knickerbockers (for Walter had not yet taken to the kilt as a regular garb, and wore it only on dress occasions), sweater and singlet and tweed jacket, boots and thick stockings, and each carried a stick. Big Brother's was one with a large knob, that we had

hollowed out and filled with lead. I was always curious about the lead affair, and all I could get by way of an answer was 'Oh, just in case'.

That was written about the beginning of a country walk of thirty miles, when Duncan II was fifteen, and was the first of many expeditions on foot and bicycle. The walk, which was minutely and lyrically described, began and ended at Callander, and the chapter concludes with their return home by train:

Our day was done and it was getting dark when we made our way to the station. The train was waiting and we got corner seats, and I must have dozed and wakened and dozed again and half slept. The carriage was a through one to the Caley Station, and I almost staggered when we got out. It was dark, and we walked home, just to cool us down, and found our Mother out looking for us at the corner of the road, listening for footsteps. 'Eh! My laddie, my laddie'. 'Oh, Mother, I've been in heaven.'

There's not much more to tell, for only dimly do I remember being helped to wash my hands, and someone sponged my face; my boots were taken off and I heard Big say 'Let me see his feet.' 'Perfect – not a spot.' Somehow I got my night-shirt on and the Mother bent and whispered, 'Say your prayers in bed to yourself tonight.' And I fear there were no prayers said that night. I slept – and Big slept at my side.

Now – one may ask – how could a boy of less than fifteen be so sensitive to all these impressions in the one day – and how could he remember them after all these many years? Ridiculous! Not so, my friend. Remember our training. We had to go into the country and gather herbs for my father's business: yarrow, eyebright, comfrey, agrimony, wormwood, tansy, elder flowers, woundwort, hawthorn berries, to name only a few; and if out with Big Bother Walter, one saw things. He was an enthusiastic field botanist, and I was shown how a flower was made. He would watch a bee burrowing deep for honey, and coming out backwards, with his back all covered with pollen; carry home flowers and he would get out his microscope and let me see the different kinds of pollen, and make sections of stems and roots and seeds and explain it all to me. A wonderful land and I was a dry sponge. Even now I have not told you half of what I remember of that first long real walk – the birds – the grass snake – the lonely cottage – the single asphodel growing in a bog – the smell of a wood fire – the majesty of the mountains – and, above all the peace and quietness – the restfulness.

That was the first walk, and it was followed by many others, and then by bicycle rides throughout much of Scotland. It would have been a strange Scotland to us today, with unmade-up roads, trains running everywhere, frequently and on time, lonely cottages in the hills where the shepherd and his wife made the walker welcome and provided ham and eggs and fresh scones, especially if the walker had a few words of Gaelic, as Walter had. Duncan ii describes it all with great emotion, and surely if he had not become a notable herbalist, he could have been a very competent author, although perhaps of the now-despised 'kail-yard' variety.

For me, the essence of the book is best caught by the description of a walk made in 1905 from Dalmally, by Loch Awe. This time, Duncan ii was accompanied by his new wife, and they were making for Port Sonachan, ten miles from Dalmally. They came across a church:

> It was a surprise, for we had passed neither house nor croft and had not noticed it marked on the map. It was a plain stone-built affair, with a thing like an aborted steeple at one end, and inside this hung the bell, with a rope reaching to the ground. There was a small porch with a stone bench; the door had neither lock nor key – the never closed door – we lifted the sneck and walked in. A dark, dull, gloomy place this, and hardly any light filtered through the small windows, and we wondered how the worshippers could see to follow the reading and singing. Doubtless they never bothered, but with sugar-bool or pandrop under their tongues, just sat, and let the thunder of hell and damnation roll over their heads. The seats were narrow wooden contraptions

with high straight backs, and nary a sign of cushion or pad, while the preacher stood at a raised reading-desk at the far end, with a seat for the precentor right under him; and wooden chairs, eight of them, for the choir, ranged round him in a half circle. There were four oil lamps standing on tall brass rods, another hanging above the reading-desk suspended from the roof, and the smell was of dry rot and mice. We sat there maybe fifteen minutes, and knew a strange peace. Inishail Church – the place of rest. In all truth, a place of worship for tired hearts and wearied bodies; a place of refreshment to the soul. What kind of worshippers came here? Did they come barefooted, carrying their Sunday boots over their arms, and putting them on at the kirk door? Did the old wives have a clean white hankie, with a sprig of rosemary or southernwood between the leaves of their Book? Did the shepherds bring their dogs? Could the boys see the girls? Did the minister preach the Gospel of Love and Peace and Contentment? To our mind's eye came the ancient hill man, short trimmed white beard, clean-shaved stiff upper lip, blue in the eye, wearing the square hard felt Sunday hat. We heard his loud amens, his groanings in the prayers, his restless movements when the preacher stumbled at the name of the father-in-law of Hezikiah; we saw his old lady nudge him as she whispered 'Not so loud, Lachlan.' The old lady with her rosy face and high cheek bones, wearing her Sunday bonnet and long white shawl, and later we heard them going over the heads of the sermon and expounding them still further. The praying mothers of great men – what does not Scotland owe these mothers? And so we left this Sanctuary of Rest and passed out into the sunlight.

A little later, Duncan II wrote about his vasculum:

Have you ever carried a vasculum – the long deep oval japanned tin box of the botanist? You can carry it by its end handle, or sling it over your shoulder by a strap. Mine was pretty full, not with plants, but food – our boiled ham made into sandwiches, a bottle of milk and two cups, bananas, greengages, Miss Macgregor's home-made scones and black currant jam.

Do you know the smell of an ancient vasculum – flowers, roots, leaves, earth, mould, moss, honey, bog-myrtle, wild thyme – all blended and indescribable. But, strange to say, this extraordinary mixture of smells never imparts itself to any food that you may be carrying in the old tin box. Maybe that's not quite true, for the food has a faint flavour of all and everything that has ever been carried in that box – all blended into one heavenly ambrosial delight. At any rate, mine had and has, and it grows more and more mellow with every fresh journey and new dent that it gets...But the opening of the old vasculum gave us another keek into the Garden of Content and, doubtless, one of the far islands was the *Tir-nan-og* – Land of Perpetual Youth – foolish dream – for only to a few of the very blessed is given the opening of the portal to the Land of Heart's Desire.

By the turn of the century, the herbal partnership of Duncan and his two sons was obviously prospering, and the family had moved several rungs up the social ladder. The selling of herbs, and the use of herbs in healing was both successful and profitable. Duncan II has described something of life at Ruby Villa in the early years of the 20th century. Breakfast was served at 7.30 on weekdays, and then, with the breakfast table still uncleared, the whole household, family, maids and 'even the washerwoman' sat round the table and lifted up their voices in a psalm. The Father (Duncan himself) read a Chapter and offered up prayers, then the day's work began, and Duncan II, the junior partner, opened the shop by 8.30.

The days were long and full. The three qualified herbalists were kept busy seeing patients, prescribing and dispensing the medications. In the basement tinctures had to be manufactured from the fresh or dried herbs, creams and ointments mixed, tablets rolled and capsules filled.

By that time, many of the medicines were made up into packages, with explanatory leaflets pasted on. Extensive correspondence had to be dealt with, and mail orders posted off to many countries. Windows needed to be dressed, and the shop premises kept well-decorated and clean. One of the windows was usually decorated by a display of the letters received from all over the world, and one of them was addressed simply: The Herbalists, Edinburgh, Scotland. Closing time was 9 pm on week days, and 10 pm on Saturdays, and even when the doors were closed, people were still standing in line to collect their medicines. It was a hard life, but surely a satisfying one.

Duncan, with his great white beard, ruddy cheeks and patriarchal appearance was still in the shop virtually every day, and it appears that he was the herbalist most patients asked to talk to. The herb gathering expeditions continued, and on one visit to the north, in 1901, Duncan climbed Ben Nevis, together with son Walter, who had some connection with the Observatory then on the summit of the Ben. For a man of seventy-one, that was a considerable feat.

As the business and practice grew, the premises at Bristo Place were transformed into a truly magnificent example of late-Victorian workmanship. Polished mahogany, gleaming brass and shining glass containers graced the shop, and a consulting room was a place of quietness and comfort. No longer did the patients have to discuss their ailments over the counter, no doubt to the delectation of those awaiting their turn.

The receipt for this work of transformation is still kept by Napiers. The work was done by John Lennox, Joiner, of Richmond Place, Edinburgh. Beautifully written on a page seemingly torn from an account book, the receipt details the work done and the material supplied between 5 September and 7 November 1878. Seven hundred and fifty-four hours of work, presumably by tradesmen, cost £28:16:11d, at the rate of ninepence-halfpenny per hour. There was also 355 hours spent in polishing, at threepence-halfpenny per hour, presumably by boys or apprentices, for a total of £4:17: 8½d. Those were the rates charged to the customer: one does rather wonder how much the men were paid. The total cost was £56:11:6½d plus six shillings for six gross of screws, with apparently a discount of £1: 17:6½d for payment of cash when the invoice was presented.

It must have seemed like an awful lot of money at the time, but the results were quite beautiful. They continued to grace the premises at Bristo Place for over a hundred years, until the last of the Napier dynasty died in 1978, and the business passed, at least temporarily, into the hands of those perhaps less appreciative of the beauty of solid wood, fine workmanship and history.

There are still records of one particular medical problem effectively dealt with by Napiers. This was tapeworm, a problem rarely encountered today, but one apparently common in Victorian Scotland. Duncan records some of his successes with this, and amongst the few remaining mementoes of those early days there are still glass jars containing the results.

It seems that in the last years of the 19th century, an American visitor to Scotland learned of the herbalist's success in dealing with tapeworm, and took back home with him some packets of the medicine. He treated his friends successfully, and was so impressed with the results that he wrote a letter to the newspapers about it, and the letter was reproduced widely throughout the United States. The result was that Napiers received many hundreds of letters, each containing a dollar bill, asking for a packet of the treatment. The medication was the pulverised seeds of *Embelia ribes*, a herb grown in India, taken fasting in the morning, mixed with milk, and followed by a purgative, usually castor oil. The worm was apparently killed by the herb, and then expelled with the aid of the castor oil. It all sounds very unpleasant, but the coiled results in the glass jars show that it was effective. As Duncan wrote: 'It was forty eight feet long, with the head of a young serpent.'

The years passed, and the business of Duncan Napier & Sons continued to prosper. However, the skies of Europe were clouding with conflict, and in 1914 the War began. In early 1915, Duncan II joined the army, and served in France until 1918. Sadly, he was badly gassed and never recovered his health. Eventually he was bed-ridden, and in 1956 he died, as another casualty of that great slaughter.

Duncan II had volunteered for the army. Conscription did not begin until 1916, and he was a married man of 35 with a young family. He need not have volunteered, but he did of his own free will. One wonders why.

Contemporary accounts of the period describe the social pressures on men to join the armed forces. In the early days of that incredible slaughter, the war seemed to be regarded as a brief holiday from the workaday world, and young men queued to be allowed to take part. The country and the Empire needed them, and they responded with all the enthusiasm of youth. Later, as the reality of those awful killing fields became obvious, joining the armed forces came to be seen as a duty, not a holiday, and as a way of repaying the country for what it had done for them. Tales, most of them fabricated, of German atrocities filled the press, and the solders and sailors and airmen were convinced, many of them, that they were defending everything they held dear against the hordes of Prussian barbarism. As the first flood of volunteers disappeared into the darkness of those Flanders fields, increasing pressure was applied to all men to play their part. Brigades of mainly comfortable middle-aged women handed out the White Feather of cowardice to all the civilian men of military age that they met.

Just which pressures influenced Duncan II we do not know, but off he went, and came back four years later a broken man, with lungs ruined by poison gas. No longer could he stalk the glens and bens of the land he loved so passionately.

The business had to continue. Duncan himself was an old man, and although still vigorous, could no longer work the long hours of the past. The whole burden fell on Andrew, and it was heavy. Wartime shortages and regulations increased the burden. Understandably, the government gave little priority to the import of herbs for civilian use. Inevitably, bureaucracy controlled whatever was available. The collection of native herbs was more essential than ever, and there was no way Andrew could cope on his own. Indeed, it could well have been the stress of all those problems that led to Andrew's early death in 1916, after 46 years of practice.

Big Brother Walter stepped in. Unselfishly, he gave up his academic career, and became a full time herbalist, tutored by his father.

That complex man Walter was a widely-known figure even before he joined the family business, and remained well-known until his death. Like his father Duncan, Walter had many interests apart from herbalism. Always wearing the kilt, he was an acknowledged authority on Highland Dress, and in all of Scotland there is no subject, except perhaps religion, more liable to cause

dissension than that! But if Walter Glendinning Napier pronounced judgement on some such arcane matter as who should be
allowed to wear a fur sporran, that was considered to be final.

Walter was one of the founders of the Scottish Society, and a
very well-known lecturer on all things Scottish. His lantern lectures
on The Road To The Isles were especially popular, and he was glad
to deliver them anywhere for any good cause. His greatest hobby,
though, was philately – the collection of postage stamps – and he
was a founder member of the Scottish Philatelic Society.

Towards the end of the war, when all the romance and glam-
our, had perished in the mud of Flanders, together with so many
of the young men, Duncan, an old man by now, wrote a long,
moving letter to his son Duncan, somewhere in that morass of
death and misery. It is the letter of an old man, and the handwriting, once so clear and vigorous, has degenerated to a scrawl.
Duncan wrote of his early youth and his struggles to become a
herbalist, and of how successful herbalism had been, and could be
again, in curing illness. There is the impression that Duncan was
encouraging his son to persist, and to return to a bright future.
Perhaps he had in mind the wartime propaganda slogan of
'Through mud and blood to the green fields beyond.'

Well, Duncan II went through the mud and the blood, and did
reach the green fields of peace. He resumed his practice together
with his father and brother Walter, but never again was he able to
take delight in long walks through the hills or cycling in the
Highlands. His lungs were ruined by poison gas, and his health
slowly deteriorated until eventually he was confined to his bed,
another victim of the war he had joined so enthusiastically.

The death of Andrew Nelson in 1916 had left the whole burden of the business and the practice on Walter Glendinning and his
aged father Duncan. There is one rather touching account of
working in the Bristo Place shop during those years. Eva, daughter of Andrew Napier, (and thus sister of Charles Napier, who
painted the portrait of Duncan), joined the staff in 1917. Young
men, of course, were scarce: the war called them and women had
to take their place in many civilian occupations. Years later, in
1977, Eva told a little of her time in Napiers:

I started to work in father's shop in the year 1917. He was very reluctant to employ me, saying 'The shop is not the place for any woman'. Up to that time only boys had helped in the shop. But it was war-time, my father's brother was away in the army, and I was very keen to lend a hand.

I left every day by tram from my home in Greenhill Gardens, changing at Tollcross. I seem to remember the fare being one penny or thereabouts. Bristo Place was a very quiet street in those days, and most vehicles were still horse-drawn.

The shop was always crammed full with customers despite the long opening hours from 9 am to 9 pm from Mondays to Fridays and from 9 am to 10 pm on Saturdays. Most were poor people who found the medicines cheaper than those obtained from the doctor. They were quite happy to stand and wait in the shop for half an hour or more.

The most popular remedies were lobelia for coughs, and skull-cap, a stimulant, for chills. Both cost 7 1/2d a bottle. Ointments could be bought for 3d. Threadworm was a common complaint among children then. Napier's had a powder for this which I had to weigh out on delicate scales and then package. None of the cures were pre-packaged as they are today.

People also came to the shop for medical advice. Grandfather stood at one counter and Father at the other. Often they favoured different remedies for the same ailment! The doctors of course didn't much like all this – they regarded the cheaper medicines as unfair competition! Napier's had no need to advertise because people recommended the cures to one another.

I never served in the shop, but worked at fetching and carrying, weighing powders and bottling medicines. I remember well the Pulmonary Lozenges which were kept on the counter and were a constant temptation to me to treat as sweeties. I recall also that New Year's Day was the only time the shop was closed apart from Sundays. But later the Government introduced a half-day closure for all shops. I also remember postcards of Duncan Napier which were given away free to customers and also sent with the medicines that went abroad.

I have always taken many of Napier's remedies myself and I am in the best of health at ninety-one!

That observant young woman, not a herbalist herself, noted one interesting thing. Two well-trained herbalists frequently prescribed different remedies for what seemed to be the same complaint. In fact, very properly, the herbalists were treating the illness, and not simply the complaint, which was probably no more than a symptom of the true illness, and which was different with each patient, although the complaint, the symptom, was the same.

Duncan Scott Napier, the founder of the business in 1860, died in 1921. That remarkable man had reached his ninety-first year, and by dint of great effort and courage, had climbed out of circumstances of poverty, ignorance and misery to achieve nation-wide recognition as a medical herbalist and healer. He had established a successful business, and had seen his family rise well up the social scale. For sixty years he practised his vocation, and was the last of the old school of herbalists who travelled the country collecting his herbs, and growing them himself in his own large garden. He watched the times change, but he never changed his convictions. Nor was he ever slow in declaring and defending those convictions. Duncan's funeral, at Grange Cemetery, was attended by a large crowd, not only of his many friends and colleagues, but also many whom he had helped in sickness. They all came to pay their last respects to a remarkable man.

The last of the Napier dynasty received his introduction to the business at the age of three months. This was John Robertson Napier, the youngest son of Duncan II. His mother brought him to the shop one day in 1914, plumped him on the counter and proudly noted that there were three generations of Napiers in the shop that day, Grandfather Duncan, father Duncan, and John Robertson.

Like his father before him, and also like his uncle Walter, John was educated at George Watson's College, but then went on to serve an apprenticeship as a chemist, and then to the School of Pharmacy in Edinburgh.

It was perhaps pre-ordained that John would become a medical herbalist and inherit the business at Bristo Place. However, his daughter Lynda insists that herbalism was by no means his first desire. Rather, he really wanted to be a forester. However, it was to herbalism that he became firmly attached, and in 1936 he formally joined the business, and became a partner with his father.

The list of John's qualifications is long and impressive: Fellow of the Medical Register of Consultant Herbalists: Fellow of the British Medical Herbalist Union (he was made a Fellow in both of those bodies in recognition of his long and distinguished services to herbalism): Member of the National Institute of Medical Herbalists: Member of the British Medical Herbalists, and finally, as a business man and not a herbalist, a Fellow of the British Society of Commerce.

John played rugby at school, and later for George Watson's Old Boys. However, apart from his herbalism, he was perhaps best known as a keen Scout. He and several other Old Watsonians organised a Scout troop for poor boys – perhaps 'disadvantaged' in today's parlance – and the lads knew him as 'Tiger Tim' after he made a spectacular jump across a burn at one of their camps. In 1939 he was appointed aide-de-camp at a World Scout Moot in Crieff in Central Scotland.

Like his father, John was also a keen cyclist, and travelled far in the Highlands. His machine was always heavily laden with bags of fresh herbs on the homeward journey. The increasing growth of Edinburgh, and the pollution of the land by modern agriculture, meant that most of the areas where the Napiers had collected their herbs locally for a hundred years could no longer be used: the herbs had disappeared from there, but still flourished in the Highlands.

As a boy, and a youth, John spent much time in the Bristo Place shop, and by the time he joined the business in 1936, aged 22, was already well acquainted with the principles and practice of herbalism. He could have had no better tutor than his father Duncan II.

Once again, the Napier principle of being apprenticed to the profession was being followed, as it had with John's father and Uncle Walter. It is a principle still followed by the renascent Napiers of Edinburgh.

However, a long period of peaceful practice was not for John.

As with his father, war intervened. Again, like his father, John promptly volunteered, and joined the Royal Navy Patrol Service.

He had been to sea before. The father of one of his friends owned trawlers plying out of Leith, and John and his friend had spent some happy holidays working on them as deckhands. Those very trawlers, and many others, were promptly requisitioned for wartime work as anti-submarine patrol boats.

Coal-fired and unarmoured, lit by oil lamps, slow, and equipped only with the lightest and oldest of guns, their one virtue was perhaps their seaworthiness. They had spent long hard years trawling in Scottish waters, and could face any weather.

John volunteered on a Wednesday, had his medical examination on Thursday, and sailed on Friday, enrolled as an Asdic operator. Asdic, or Anti-Submarine Detection Investigation Committee, now known as sonar, is that device we have all heard in a hundred films about the war. Its characteristic regular 'Ping. Ping' has marked many a tense moment in those films. It did in reality too, as the note of the returning echo denoted a lurking submarine.

So those young men went to sea. They had no uniforms, but eventually these were provided, in the shape of ten armbands, marked 'RN By courtesy of the Admiralty'. They had little else, either. There is a letter sent by a lady to John's future wife Kathleen thanking her for sending high necked blue woollen pullovers for the use of the men at sea, and asking for blankets made from brightly coloured squares of hand knitting, 'which cheered up the bunks'.

Those battered old trawlers patrolled the North Sea, and saw much action, protecting as best they could the convoys of ships on which so much depended. A little later, after the terrible defeat which culminated in the evacuation of what was left of the British Army, and much of the French, from the beaches of Dunkirk, John was engaged in patrolling the English Channel.

This he always described as the most difficult and dangerous time. Equipped by now with barrage balloons to discourage dive bombers, they did their best to guard the convoys. One such convoy of 22 ships lost thirteen of them.

Mines, e-boats, dive bombers and cannon fire from the French coast were everyday experiences. A little later, based at Belfast, the old trawlers patrolled the Western Approaches.

Promoted to a Higher Submarine Detector, John was transferred to a new vessel, *HMS Rosalind*, and she was meant for service in the Far East. Sailing alone, this trawler-type patrol boat went far out into the Atlantic before rounding South Africa, on to Aden, India and Ceylon before reaching her station off the Seychelles. Together with another patrol boat, the *Rosalind* was there to protect the twenty-nine islands of the Seychelles from the Japanese Navy. Since the four battleships of that navy had just sunk the British battleships *Prince of Wales* and *Repulse*, their protection would not have been very effective. As John said later, their only hope, if the Japanese had appeared, would have been to pray for fog.

By now a Leading Seaman, John had his tonsils taken out by an operation in Durban, and that must have been a strange experience for him, a well-qualified herbalist, who would certainly have known how to cure himself, if only he had access to the dispensary at Bristo Place. At one point, John was given a commission and posted to a battleship, but that did not last long. He resigned his commission, and returned to the patrol boats.

In early 1944, he was returned to Britain, and on his leave, married Kathleen Mairi McLean. They had first met when Kathleen was a young girl singing in the choir of John's church. John and his patrol boat continued service until November 1945, when he was finally released, and returned to his business and practice.

His father, Duncan II, had continued all through the war to hold the business together, as best he could, in the face of steadily declining health due to his gassing in the First War. By 1945, about ten people were employed in the business.

John's children, Kenneth MacLean Napier, born in 1946, and Lynda Mairi Napier, born in 1948, both still vividly recall holidays as far away as the Outer Hebrides, largely spent in collecting herbs, eyebright, St. John's wort, meadowsweet, yarrow, hawthorn berries, all essential for use in the practice, and which had to be gathered at the right times and from unpolluted areas.

At that time, John was one of only four qualified herbalists in Scotland. Apart from his apprenticeship as a chemist and his qualification from the School of Dispensary and Pharmacy, he had served the requisite five years apprenticeship with his father, studied the art of herbalism for three years, and then passed his examinations in London. There could be no doubt about the depth of his knowledge, and furthermore he had absorbed the essential diagnostic skills from all the time he had spent with his father and uncle.

John Napier lived a very busy life. A professional qualified herbalist, he was never content to be just that. He even trained and qualified as a Member of the Pelman Institute, that rather strange body designed for 'The Scientific Development of Mind and Memory'. An enthusiastic car driver, he passed the test of the Institute of Advanced Motorists, and joined the motorised section of the Special Constabulary and served them for fifteen years. Promoted and decorated in the service, he was made a Knight Commander and a full member of the International Police Association.

Like his uncle Walter, John was an enthusiast for all things Scottish, and wore the kilt regularly, as an active member of both the Scottish Society and the St. Andrew's Society. An enthusiastic Rotarian, he took an active part in all the charitable activities of his Rotary Club of Central Edinburgh. He was the youngest Deacon to be appointed by his Church, and was an Elder of the Church for many years.

He did indeed carry a heavy load of work, duty and charity. One must wonder whether he grossly overloaded himself, and whether that contributed to his sudden death. Walking home one wintry night in February 1978, John collapsed and died in the road just a hundred yards or so from his house.

Changing Times

Before he died so untimely a death, John Napier had the satisfaction of organising the Centenary celebrations for Napiers, Herbalists of Edinburgh.

That was in 1960, and the main event was a dinner at an Edinburgh hotel. It was a grand affair, with the main speeches given by John and his brother Dick, a GP in Norwich. Unfortunately, there is no record of their speeches, but the programme shows what must have been a fine evening of eating, speeches, song and dancing. It was attended by a large number of colleagues from John's many interests, and by representatives of many firms John dealt with.

John certainly had had many lessons in the arcane art of publicity by that time, and the Centenary celebration produced much interest in the press, and, of course, that generated much business.

John also wrote a booklet, *A Century of Herbalism at Napiers*. After sketching Napier's story, it listed and described many of the remedies then being produced by the business. It makes interesting reading, especially when compared with the Napiers catalogue of today.

Referring to Duncan Napier's first product, Lobelia Cough Syrup, for example, John wrote:

This Lobelia Syrup has been used by us for over 100 years with the most surprising and happy success, both in old and young as a special and specific remedy for chest complaints.

In Bronchitis, Asthma, Difficulty of Breathing, and long-standing coughs, it loosens the phlegm from the bronchial tubes, thus rendering the cough easy and allowing the patient freedom of breathing during the day, and the benefit of a night's rest. For Cough accompanying Inflammation and Pleurisy, it renders special benefit by detaching the mucus and inducing a healthier condition. For recent and common cough it gives almost immediate relief. For Children it possesses similar advantages. It is a specific for Croup (a dose every fifteen minutes until relieved). It is our first choice of medicines during Whooping Cough, as it shortens the spasm and eases the cough, maintains the appetite and prevents serious after-effects.

In Napiers' current catalogue, the Lobelia Syrup still figures, of course, but is tersely described simply as 'Napiers famous bronchial expectorant, using Duncan Napier's original recipe.' This terseness is not because the herbalist of today does not believe in the efficacy of Lobelia Syrup – they would probably endorse John's words. Rather, the regulations governing advertisements and publicity today are so strict that no claims can be made for the effectiveness of herbal products.

Even if the law permitted, Napiers of today would not advertise Herbal Smoking Mixture in the way that John Napier thought it right to do in his 1960 Centenary booklet:

> The Bristo Brand was introduced by us many years ago to meet the demand for a Smoking Mixture, devoid of hurtful results to the nerves or digestion. The immense success of this Mixture induces us to make known its benefits, as it can be smoked with perfect freedom by those who suffer from a weak heart or failing eyesight. There is nothing poisonous or deleterious in the process of manufacture; the leaves and flowers are selected and combined with rare taste and perfect knowledge, producing in the combination a unique Smoking Mixture, giving the enjoyment of a smoke – the soothing relief and satisfaction.
>
> Its flavour when smoking is pleasant, its aroma agreeable, while no harsh taste is left in the mouth.
>
> It also possesses medicinal advantages. The inhalation of the smoke exerts a balsamic and soothing influence over the lungs and respiratory organs, clearing colds in the head, removing phlegm, and giving freedom of breathing in Asthma, Bronchitis etc.
>
> Recommended to Old People to assist their breathing.

In the previous chapter, the lady who assisted in Napiers during the Great War said that they had no need to advertise, that word of mouth recommendations were enough. Well, the times they were indeed a-changing. Advertising in the time of John Napier was essential to maintain and grow the business.

Shortly after the War in which John was so involved, the great National Health Service was established. It was established in the face of almost universal opposition from the medical professions and their organisations. 'Socialised Medicine', they called it, and they fought it long and hard. Aneurin Bevan, the Government Minister responsible for establishing the NHS, recorded that he finally got the consultants to accept it only by 'stuffing their mouths with gold.'

There was no charge in those halcyon days for any item prescribed by a doctor, and prescriptions were handed out freely for everything from packets of cotton wool to wigs and aspirin tablets. Ask for it, and you got it, and there is no doubt that the system was exploited by many. There is equally no doubt that many in the medical professions hoped to sabotage the service by making it impossibly expensive to the Government. In attempting to limit the expense, the Government finally introduced a charge, of sixpence, for filling prescriptions, and as a result Aneurin Bevan resigned in protest at what he regarded as an abandonment of the vital principle of the NHS, that it should be free and available to all, and that it should be paid for by central government and financed by a National Insurance paid by all employees and employers.

Herbalists and all other alternative practitioners were of course excluded from the NHS. Their patients still had to pay for consultations and medicine, and inevitably the herbalists lost a great deal of business. Why visit a herbalist and pay half a crown for a consultation and seven pence half-penny for a bottle of cough mixture when your GP would happily write a prescription and you got the cough mixture for free.

It seemed at first that the whole structure of herbalism might collapse, and with it the very large international trade in herbs. The biggest importer and dealer in herbs and herbal preparations at that time was probably Potters. They had a large manufacturing plant upriver from London, and a regular service of lighters carried the raw materials from London Docks. They had to close that plant, with the loss of six hundred jobs. Nor were they alone in having such a problem. All over the country the herbal business contracted.

In that climate, John Napier had to adapt, and learn how to use effective advertising and publicity. He learned fast and well, and undoubtedly it was those new-learned skills, plus his reputation as a healer and a well-known figure that enabled Napiers to survive. Many others did not. Amongst his many other activities John was always ready to lecture any audience on herbalism, and no doubt that helped the business over some difficult years.

It was not all herbalism and hard work, though. John has recounted how he was once asked to supply a large amount of dried tamarinds as a tonic for the elephants in Edinburgh Zoo. On another occasion, a bird fancier from Fife wanted a cure for a favourite canary which had croup and could no longer sing. A few spoonfuls of comfrey extract restored it to health and full song. A hectic day was once spent powdering dried nettles to feed mosquitoes at the Research Department of Edinburgh University.

When John died, his widow, Kathleen, had perforce to take over control of the business, and this she did with much energy and initiative. But of course she was not a herbalist, and efforts were made by professional friends of John to keep the practice going. Eric Robson, a highly qualified and successful herbalist in Newcastle travelled regularly to Edinburgh to treat patients, and Helen Flucker, a well-advanced student of John's, did what she could.

In many ways at that time, the legal position of herbalism in the UK was uncertain and ambiguous. The law seemed to forbid its practice, except under the direction and control of an allopathic doctor, and yet in fact the law was rarely applied.

Back at the inception of the NHS, Aneurin Bevan was able to justify his decision to exclude herbalists from the service by pointing out that there was no single organisation representing them, and that the vast majority of herbalists then practising had no formal qualification or training. There were perhaps as many as 1,500 herb shops then still in existence, and the owners, by and large, had no formal training. There were only 500 qualified herbalists organised in any professional body, with regular courses of education and clinical training. Furthermore, the qualified herbalists still displayed all the same fissiparous tendencies that had so weakened them in the past. Rarely could they speak with one voice, even when their whole future was at stake.

At different times, and sometimes simultaneously, there was the British Institute of Organic Medicine, the National Association of Medical Herbalists, the British Herbalists' Union, the British Health Freedom Society, the Society of Physical Medicine, and the Congress of Natural Healing. It was hardly surprising that the Ministry of Health, even had it wanted to do so, could find no single organisation which represented herbalism.

Perhaps there was also a psychological or emotional problem within the government. In Nazi Germany, even from its earliest days in power, herbal and other folk medicines were strongly encouraged. They were claimed to be Aryan, and thus must be nurtured. From Hitler himself, and his deputy Hess, the word went out, and herbalism and research into herbal remedies boomed. Universities and medical schools were instructed to establish Chairs in Pharmacognosy – the science of the description of plants – and what was already a considerable industry in producing medical plants and remedies was encouraged as a patriotic duty.

And it was not only Nazi Germany that, in the 1930s, saw a remarkable growth in alternative medicine. All over the mainland of Europe there was a great upsurge in, and use of, herbalism, homeopathy, naturopathy, yoga, osteopathy, and exercise classes. The present writer well recalls the British Womens' League of Health and Beauty, under its formidable leader Prunella Stack. Sports fields all over the country, and every exercise hall, were filled with young women in very tight, very short, shorts, leaping and moving gracefully as they danced. Never before had young men been so tantalised by bouncing bosoms, flashing legs, and swirling silk scarves.

Such a surging of alternative practices of course roused the allopathic medical professions to anger, and to action.

Perhaps partly because Nazi Germany, the enemy, had adopted herbal medicine so wholeheartedly, and had so distorted it into the belief in Aryan Supremacy, the British Parliament struck what might have been, and almost was, a fatal blow against herbalism.

In 1941, in the darkest days of the war, when the whole of western Europe, except UK, was under Nazi occupation, Parliament somehow found time to rush through a Pharmacy and Medicines Act which removed the ancient right of herbalists to supply their patients with medicines, and thus at one stroke made them illegal practitioners of medicine. It is of course significant that in Parliament more than 60 allopathic doctors were members of the House of Commons, and that the House of Lords contained a number of illustrious physicians and surgeons.

Parliament and Government were certainly not prepared for the ensuing storm of protest. Even though many of its younger members, like John Napier, were absent in the Services, the National Association of Medical Herbalists organised such a campaign of protest that assurances were received that, although the Act must remain on the Statute Book, Association members could continue to practice, and it was agreed that herbalists would be consulted about any future medical legislation. They had to be content with those assurances.

Even in such an atmosphere of uncertainty and semi-legality, herbal practitioners still failed to unite into one coherent body speaking with one voice. They did, though, begin to put their house in order, especially by organising regular training and education.

Throughout the 1940s and 1950s, the profession of herbal medicine still drifted, half illegal, and existing only because the authorities turned a blind eye to it. That must have been a difficult time for John Napier, but he kept his business and his practice afloat, moving and manipulating as various new regulations demanded, sometimes being the only qualified herbalist in the city of Edinburgh.

Time after time, the pharmaceutical industry released information on new wonder drugs. Time after time, the public was regaled with headlines about 'Breakthrough for heart patients', 'Cancer cure in sight', 'New hope for arthritis sufferers', and so on, and just as frequently the new drugs failed in practice, or produced side-effects worse than the original complaint.

Some of those side-effects were slight and transient – a touch of diarrhoea or constipation, dry eyes perhaps, or a persistent headache.

Others were serious and indeed life-threatening. By the 1960s, those illnesses actually caused by drugs prescribed by doctors seemed themselves to be a new disease, so much so that one writer, Ivan Illich, coined the expression 'iatrogenic disease' – doctor-induced disease. 'The medical establishment has become a major threat to health', he wrote, perhaps unknowingly echoing the views of Napoleon a century and a half earlier. An American Government report in 1969 stated that one seventh of all hospital days were spent in treating that newly named disease. The cost in financial terms was horrendous, and in terms of human suffering was incalculable.

In the West, the 1960s was that strange decade of Youth and Flower Power, of the invention of sex as a participatory sport, of Free Love (free of the fear of pregnancy, that is) and of loud music. Rachel Carson's book *Silent Spring* recounted the damage that pollutants were having on the environment, and forecast a near future when spring would indeed be silent because all the birds were dead of pollution. There was another tremendous upsurge of the cult of nature in all its forms, of Back to the Land, and of the 'Good Life'. So-called health food shops sprang up everywhere, books and magazines on health and nutrition proliferated, alternative and complementary treatments flourished as never before, as 'progress' was rejected and a return to 'nature' began to seem desirable, necessary and indeed inevitable. New forms of treatment appeared, from crystal healing to shiatsu. Whether effective or not, at least they were harmless, and were never regarded as a threat by the medical establishment. Herbalism, as ever, was so regarded.

In 1964, the UK Ministry of Health began drafting a new Medicines Bill. *Hansard*, the Parliamentary record, shows clearly that Ministers and their minions remembered only too well the storm of successful protest that the 1941 Bill had produced. This time, they informed the herbalists' bodies of what they proposed.

What they proposed was in fact a catastrophe for herbal medicine. The proposals meant the end of herbalism, and of the manufacture of herbal medicines. Over-the-counter sales of herbal products had up to that time been relatively uncontrolled, except for those products regarded as poisonous – chiefly herbs that could be used as abortificants. Again, it was proposed that herbal remedies should be sold only in pharmacies and under the control of pharmacists.

It was proposed to set up a Committee to evaluate all medicines for safety and efficacy. Naturally, it was a Committee of doctors and pharmacists. They were hardly likely to approve of traditional herbal products.

Once again, the profession of herbalism, and the associated herbal industry, together with the proliferating health food retailers, had to fight for their professional lives. This time they were determined to present a united front. The , the Society of Herbalists, manufacturers and retailers joined together in the British Herbal Medicine Association, and entered into discussions with the Ministry as one body.

Surprise, surprise! They were no longer treated with the disdain of the past. If the disparate forces of herbalism, in 1941, in the midst of a war which was going badly, could produce such a storm of protest, what could they do in 1964, when the forces of 'natural living' were so much more vocal, so many in number, so united, and so much more able and willing to protest at any attack upon what was regarded as a basic freedom?

In their approach to the Ministry, the representatives of the British Herbal Medical Association were not only warmly received, but received immediate assurances that the Minister himself had made it clear that there was no desire or intention to injure or kill herbalism. Furthermore, the civil servants had been instructed that 'measures must be found to preserve the rights of persons who wished to undertake herbal treatment or to purchase herbal remedies'.

That was indeed fine so far as it went, but it left one major question. Was the Ministry going to insist that herbal remedies undergo the same testing for safety and efficacy that new chemical drugs had to undergo? If so, that, too, would mark the end of herbalism, for such testing was horrendously expensive. It took years to complete, entailed much experimentation on animals, and was, in both theory and practice, totally opposed to the philosophy and ethos of herbalism. Nor, of course, was it in any way always effective, as the tragedies of Thalidomide and Eraldin showed.

Hearing it with the greatest relief, the Association was informed that the Ministry 'would accept as proof of safety and efficacy the fact that a herb had been in use for a long period without giving any ill-effect and presumably producing results satisfactory to the consumer.' Any herb about which a monograph appeared in any standard reference book and was not poisonous would be acceptable.

Although by no means the sort of ringing declaration that his scribes had produced for Henry VIII in his Herbalists' Charter, those ministerial assurances were certainly acceptable and helpful. However, as with so many assurances given by civil servants and politicians, there were a number of weasel words – words that were not defined, and could bear several meanings. What was 'a long period' in which herbs had been used safely? Was it ten years? Or was it perhaps a thousand years? What was 'a standard reference book', and who would define it?

To the herbalists, there seemed to be only one way to be certain of meeting that last requirement, and that was to themselves produce such a reference book. This they determined to do, and the result is the *British Herbal Pharmacopoeia*.

A committee of distinguished scientists and herbal practitioners was established to write the monographs, to read and evaluate all written material, and to ensure that there was a sound basis for the continued use by herbalists of all herbs in general use.

A unique publication, the *British Herbal Pharmacopoeia* became, and remains, the basic reference book for herbal practitioners in the English-speaking world. Regularly updated in its loose-leaf form, it is hardly bedtime reading even for the most dedicated herbalist. But it is a standard reference book, and does contain monographs and thus meets in all respects the requirements of the Ministry.

Whilst the Scientific Committee was labouring to produce the *Pharmacopoeia*, the minions of the Ministry of Health were beavering away to produce the Parliamentary Bill. Within the herbal community there were those who worried that no government could be trusted, that no Ministry so influenced by the medical professions and the pharmaceutical industry would willingly safeguard the profession of herbalism and the industry of producing herbal medicines.

Of course, that cynicism was justified. When the proposed Bill was published, it contained provisions that would have totally outlawed herbalism. The use by herbalists of herbal tinctures, pills, creams, ointments, pesssaries, suppositories and capsules was forbidden. The only form in which herbs could be administered was fresh, dried or powdered, and they must be mixed with no non-herbal constituent but water. A herbalist would not be allowed to make house calls, and any refill prescriptions (if there could have been such a thing) could only be collected by the patient himself, even if that patient was confined to bed. Worst of all, perhaps, was a vast reduction in the number of herbs that a herbalist could use. So much, then, for the weasel words of the Minister and his bureaucrats.

As ever, though, those set in power over us were not prepared for the hurricane they provoked. The whole united might of the herbal world, practitioners, manufacturers, retailers and satisfied consumers inundated Parliament and government with protests. The community at large, perhaps wearied by yet another example of nanny government, was determined to support their ancient right to use herbal medicine if they wished to. It was said that no other public campaign designed to influence Parliament had ever been so intense and widespread.

Step by step, yard by yard, herb by herb, the Men from the Ministry retreated under attack. (The military analogy is justified: the herbal profession was fighting for its life, and its users for their health and their freedom of choice.) When the final form of the Bill was published in 1968, almost none of the proposed restrictions were included. A few herbs were restricted in their use, and a few (which no qualified herbalist would have used anyway), were forbidden.

The herbalists had won their battle, but the manufacturers of herbal products did suffer. They found themselves subject to the same regulations as the pharmaceutical industry. Much increased documentation – the paper work beloved of bureaucrats – was demanded. Stricter controls were placed on laboratories and quality control. But each existing proprietary medicine did receive a License of Right, although they all had to be re-registered, new licences applied for, and labels re-worded. It was enormously expensive for them, and some smaller firms were driven out of business.

However, the manufacturers had won their main point. The original proposal had been that proprietary herbal remedies could be sold only in a pharmacy and under the control of a pharmacist. Their main market in fact was with the health food shops, and in the Bill the right to sell them there was confirmed.

John Napier had of course been deeply involved in this campaign, as a member of the Committee of the British Herbal Medicine Association, and as Treasurer of the Association for six years. It could not have been easy for him to leave his one-man practice for repeated lobbying visits and Committee meetings in London. But John had ever thrived on hard work. With the success of the campaign, however, he could no longer produce his tinctures and other medicines in a gloomy cellar, using oak barrels and stirring them with a stick, as his father, his uncles and his grandfather had done. The process of modernisation had begun, and it was in fact all for the best. Higher standards in manufacture, a more hygienic system, and greater scientific knowledge were all now required, and this is bound to increase the faith of the public in the modern version of the ancient art of healing with herbs.

The other great benefit to come out of that astonishing campaign to preserve herbalism is the *British Herbal Pharmacopoeia*. It was the first of its kind in the West, and remains by far the best, and is an invaluable reference book for all who practice herbalism.

That 1968 Medicines Bill did mark the end of one traditional form of herbalism, and that was the backstreet herbalist, usually with a stock of dusty herbs and no formal training. In a sense, it was sad to see him go. Although by now anachronistic, he was in fact the direct descendant of all those domestic and folk healers of old who had provided the only medical help for the mass of people over many centuries. But he was a stage-coach in an era of express trains and jet air-liners. There was no way he could possibly achieve the required standards of learning and hygiene, and on the whole those standards were beneficial and indeed essential to the continued profession of herbalism. So the back street herbalist disappeared into the mists of history, and the perhaps considerable amount of pragmatic knowledge he possessed went with him. The Wise Woman, the bone-setter, the monk-herbalist had already gone. With the disappearance of the back street herbalist, herbal medicine entered a new and surely better phase, a phase of trained professionalism.

Napiers Resurgent

O, mickle is the powerful grace that lies in herbs...

Shakespeare: *Romeo and Juliet*

The years following John Napier's death in 1978 were a period of great difficulty and decline for both the business and the practice.

Kathleen Napier, John's widow, did everything she possibly could to hold things together, but all her hard work was really not enough. Without a resident qualified herbalist, much of the shop's trade disappeared, since there were no prescriptions to be filled. The occasional visit by a herbalist always saw the waiting room full, but that by no means made up for the many days when the waiting room door was locked. A loyal staff, trained by John, together with Kathleen's children, certainly supported Kathleen, but the bulk of the work, and the management of the business, was her responsibility. She still gathered some herbs, dressed the windows, hand printed show-cards, and decorated the premises with flowers from her own garden.

Sadly, but surely inevitably, Kathleen decided that she had no alternative: she must sell the business, the practice, or what remained of it, and the premises.

In the years before his death, John Napier had worked very hard, and spent much money, to acquire the necessary licences for many of the products devised by himself, his father, his uncle and his grandfather over the previous hundred years. Many of the products had to be modified to meet the new regulations, and in fact John tested many of them on himself. Those Licenses were a very valuable asset of the business, and must have been a considerable factor in convincing the purchaser to make an offer which was acceptable to Kathleen.

Those purchasers were already in the herbal business in the south of England, and could not have found it easy to operate such a complex acquisition as Napiers at such a distance.

New owners of course brought new ideas. Perhaps with the determination to 'modernise' the premises, they dismantled and disposed of the polished mahogany and shining brass fittings of the shop and consulting room, and replaced them with aluminium and plastic. As it happened, an Edinburgh museum had already expressed great interest in the original shop and consulting room, so lovingly installed by Duncan Napier a hundred years earlier, and had gone to the length of preparing a room in which to install them. Had that happened, the museum would have had the only exhibit in the country of a 19th century herbal shop. But it was not to be.

As the years passed, the business went through different hands, and gradually began changing character, from being a herbalist's shop, to more and more resembling another of the increasingly common health food shops. The name of 'Napiers' was preserved, there was still a herbal dispensary and a certain amount of producing the old remedies was carried on. The once considerable mail order business withered away.

The basic problem, of course, was that there was no full-time qualified herbalist working there. No amount of over-the-counter advice from experienced but unqualified shop staff, and no amount of over-the-counter sales of packets and bottles of herbal preparations could replace the guidance of the herbalist and the prescriptions he wrote.

Eventually, the business and the premises came into the hands of Jan de Vries. Jan was then, and still is, perhaps the premier and most successful alternative practitioner in the country. Based in Ayrshire, South-west Scotland, he has clinics in various other places. A prolific and entertaining writer, he also owned a small chain of health food shops. It has never been properly explained, and it is certainly difficult to understand, how Jan ever managed to do everything he did, and do it so well. He still does.

His residence, and his main clinic, is a very large and beautiful house standing in several acres of grounds. There are several treatment rooms, and after a consultation with Jan, the patient is directed, if necessary, to one of them to receive acupuncture, osteopathy, or whatever is deemed necessary. It is quite normal for

Jan to be literally trotting along the corridor, superintending the insertion of acupuncture needles here, the manipulation of a spine there, the application of aromatherapy oils in the next cubicle.

It is not at all clear why Jan de Vries acquired the business and premises of Napiers, but certainly he was concerned that such a once integral part of Scottish herbalism was in danger of withering away completely. He had of course known John Napier well – they had fought together to defeat the 1968 attempt by the Government to kill off herbalism and other alternative treatments. However, as well as being a very successful alternative practitioner, Jan is an astute businessman, and most certainly he would have been influenced by the business potential of Napiers, as well as by the wish to preserve a vital part of herbal history.

The basic problem remained, though. There was still no resident herbalist in Napiers, and there simply was no way that Jan himself could practice there regularly and frequently. There were no qualified herbalists in Edinburgh at that time.

It is necessary here to give a little personal information. My wife and I, and our two daughters, returned to live in Scotland after about ten years spent in Wales. There, imbued with the ideas of John Seymour, we had tried to live the Good Life as small (very small) self-sufficient farmers. It was successful enough, and the living was good, but not good enough. There is no way you can be self-sufficient in modern society. You must have an income to buy the essential things that you cannot produce on the land. The sale of an occasional calf or a litter of piglets is not enough.

Fortunately, in the hills of north Pembrokeshire at that time, there was a community of Back to the Land settlers, most of them, like ourselves, flushed with enthusiasm by a close reading of John Seymour's seductive books – and the sale of those books enabled John, our neighbour, to live well on his small holding. Cottages, in various degrees of decrepitude, were then quite plentiful and reasonably cheap, and many surprised local farmers were only too delighted to sell off some of their less useful land to this influx of new peasants. Some of those peasants worked hard and successfully, co-operating in the labour of harvesting, lending each other the old and worn-out implements picked up for coppers at farm sales, exchanging half a freshly slaughtered pig for a quarter of beef. Others relapsed into, or never escaped from, a dream world of neglect and guitar playing, strange-smelling roll-ups, and endless home-brewed beer, and talking of how tomorrow they would put up that fence or muck out the byre.

Still, as John Seymour had it as the title of his first, and best, book, it was *The Fat Of The Land*. Literally so, when I think back on that diet of endless Jersey milk, cream, butter, meat of all descriptions, organic vegetables before we had heard the word 'organic', nourished as they were with an endless supply of muck from the byre and pig-pen, and limitless home-brewed beer and wines. I am astonished that all our arteries did not need a regular reaming out.

This was particularly true in my case. For many years I had been troubled by a duodenal ulcer which, although constantly painful and occasionally flaring into a real problem, never seemed to be quite bad enough for a surgeon to get interested in it. The treatment was antacid tablets and a 'soft' diet. Well, I certainly had that, in spades. Small, regular, frequent and appetising meals was the prescription, and that meant copious amounts of Jersey milk, butter, cheese, home-baked bread, home-cured bacon, fresh-caught fish and meat which never saw a butcher's slab. Perhaps John Seymour was right (although I fear he was wrong) when he argued vehemently over pints of home-brew that the arteries did not fur up if the body was worked hard. He also argued, and it was true, that you do not gain weight if you work hard enough physically. Thirty years later, living off a diet of reduced fats, reduced meats, little bread and masses of green leaves, I am three stones heavier.

But the antacids and the soft diet did not work. My old friend the ulcer grew steadily more troublesome, and eventually the doctor began to talk about exploratory operations. It so happened that a new neighbour was David Hoffmann. He had newly qualified as a herbalist, and whilst entering whole-heartedly and joyously into the free-and-easy life of our local 'hippy' society, opened a herbal clinic nearby.

Without knowing a thing about herbalism, but feeling that it seemed to be much more in tune with the ideas I espoused than were the clinical attitudes of the doctor, I decided to consult him, carrying as payment a leg of lamb and a dozen eggs. The result, I thought then, and know today, was little short of an immediate transformation. After a week of taking his prescription (a murky, evil-tasting bottle of liquid), and greatly modifying my diet, I was, for the first time in 20 years, free from pain.

My daughters watched all this with the greatest interest, and, with no parental pressure of any kind, both determined to become herbalists. Dee, the elder, first took an honours degree in Social Studies; the younger, Non, refused to waste time, as she saw it, at University, and after wandering the world for a year or so, went to the School of Herbal Medicine and Phytotherapy for their four-year full time course. After taking her degree, and also wandering the world, Dee joined her two years later.

After graduating, Non (or Chanchal as she was now called, having been given a new name by her spiritual teacher in an Indian ashram) took over a faltering, almost moribund herbal practice in Glasgow, together with another newly graduated herbalist.

In 1986, Glasgow held a marvellous Garden Festival, and amongst the many attractions was a herb garden, which Chanchal organised and nurtured. Various panels and discussions were organised, and on one of them, which was televised, Jan and Chanchal met for the first time. Jan, with all his years of experience, was an old hand at that sort of public discussion of complementary medicine; Chanchal, young and still struggling to establish herself in the world of healing, was not experienced, but her enthusiasm and an innate ability to articulate her ideas and ideals shone through.

Jan must have been impressed, for after the cameras were turned off, he offered the Napiers of Edinburgh practice to her. This was an incredible opportunity for a young herbalist. To take over a practice established over a hundred years earlier, with all its history and reputation, was the sort of thing a young herbalist could only dream about.

But it was not to be. Chanchal had very recently irrevocably committed herself to move to Vancouver, and seek to establish herself there as a qualified herbalist, in an environment much more open to the alternative, the complementary, the natural.

However, she was able to tell Jan that her elder sister, Dee, was a newly qualified herbalist, and was seeking to establish a practice, preferably in Scotland, and ideally in Edinburgh. Jan and Dee met, found that they shared ideals and principles, and Dee became the resident herbalist at Napiers of Edinburgh, the heir to its long tradition and reputation.

Although not relevant to the saga of Napiers, and really only as a proud parental interjection, it is interesting to note that, after much initial struggle, Chanchal established not only a vibrant herbal practice in Vancouver, but also the Gaia Herbal Dispensary and Clinic, with two outlets in the city. As well as being a member for several years now of various Canadian Government bodies controlling complementary medicine, she is at present also involved in a very large research programme in Oregon, investigating complementary medical treatments for cancer. And this, while maintaining her own practice in Vancouver.

So Dee opened her waiting room doors, and the patients began appearing. It was not like the old days of Duncan Napier, when it was said that patients queued along the street, but certainly it was sufficient to allow a second young herbalist, also newly qualified, to begin practising there. It was a strange situation, really. The premises were owned by Jan de Vries, the shop and dispensary by a small chain of health food stores centred in England, and the growing practice by Dee.

A very real problem was that there was only one consulting room. It was in constant use six days each week by Dee and her herbalist colleague, and there was no accommodation for the osteopath, acupuncturist and aromatherapist that Dee saw clearly must be part of a complementary clinic, and to which the two herbalists needed to refer some patients.

So negotiations were opened, and eventually, after much discussion, Dee was able to acquire the lease of the premises, and became the owner of Napiers of Edinburgh, shop, practice and that indefinable thing called goodwill.

At that time the whole operation of the shop and dispensary

was run by two redoubtable women. Between them they dressed the windows, stacked the shelves, served the customers, dispensed prescriptions, made appointments, sent out mail order orders and wholesale orders, made, bottled and packed medicines, counted the takings each night and banked the proceeds. All this in premises which although certainly clean and attractive enough for the mid-century, and efficient enough forty years earlier, were in fact hopelessly out-of-date for the late century. The plumbing system was a disaster, and the electrical system a dangerous joke.

Traditionally new brooms sweep clean, but in this case shovels, not brooms, were required. The collected detritus of generations had to be cleared, and many astonishing artefacts were discovered, not least of them Duncan Napier's original collection of tapeworms he had dislodged from their unwilling hosts. The large but crowded basement which was the store room and manufactory, had to be scraped down and painted, the shop re-organised to allow self-service for everything but certain herbal products, the dispensary totally re-built. A room behind the waiting room had long been used for making ointments and creams, and as they simmered away, the often pungent smells drifted like one of the notorious Edinburgh haars (fogs) over the waiting patients. That room was required as a new consulting room, and was totally gutted, wood-panelled, the old very high plaster ceiling lowered, and the whole lovingly decorated and equipped. On the very morning it was to be used for the first time, the old plaster ceiling fell down, bringing down the new ceiling with it. A bath had overflowed in one of the apartments above the shop. Those apartments belonged to the University, and were occupied by post-graduate students and families from places not familiar with the vagaries of Victorian plumbing. It took just one day for an extraordinary gang of joiners and shop fitters to restore the damage, although for some weeks after that, waiting patients enjoyed, if that is the right word, a nasty whiff of stale bath water and old plaster, instead of the simmering calendula ointment.

Quickly, but hardly soon enough for an impatient Dee, the premises were transformed into an attractive and reasonably efficient modern herbal shop, dispensary and clinic.

My wife and I, Dee's parents, had been much involved during that time, with shovel, scrubbing brush, paint brush, hammer and saw. We had been initiated into the strange world of the Receptionist, who juggles patients and practitioners, and tries hard to not drop either of them. We had counted pills and capsules, dispensed prescriptions, made tinctures, ointments and creams, and served customers. Perhaps the only major mistake we made was made by me. At an exhibition of alternative medicine in Glasgow, Dee had gone off to deliver a talk, leaving me in charge of the stall. A man asked for something to deal with his acne, and I sold him a jar of ointment actually meant for piles. Wrong ointment, wrong end, in fact. Surprisingly, he appeared in the shop a week later, and bought another jar of the same ointment, saying he was sure it was working. I did not enquire what it was working on.

Never one to allow any opportunity for good publicity to pass, Dee was entered into the annual competition that year, and won the accolade of Best Young Businesswoman of the Year in Edinburgh. The following year, she was entered into another competition, televised this time, and was runner-up as Best Young Business Person in Scotland. Perhaps naturally, I was convinced – still am – that she should have won.

As the time passed – actually quite a short time – other complementary practitioners used the clinic facilities, shop staff were trained, and the time had come for the parents to leave.

However, Dee entrusted me with the re-vitalisation of the mail order service, which had been almost dead for several years. Although we live on the opposite side of the country from Edinburgh, in these days of telephones, faxes and e-mail, it was no problem to do that from my own office. Since my own trade at the time was publishing, I was able to prepare and issue a mail-order catalogue, and soon trade was brisk. So brisk, in fact, that after a few years, Dee decided that the mail-order business had to be repatriated to Edinburgh, where it could be run in conjunction with a Herbal Helpline, a regular Newsletter, a web site of course, and ultimately a magazine, *HERB*. That was the first of three times that I was made redundant from Napiers, and by my own daughter, which must be something of a record. The second time was after I had launched the Newsletter, and the third after launching the magazine. However, they still find that a keen, if octogenarian eye, is required for reading the proofs of all publications.

Very shortly, as the number of practitioners increased, the demand for greater manufacturing capacity increased accordingly. The size of the premises was a corset which restricted expansion. At some time when the business was in other hands, after John Napier's death, part of the premises – once a consulting room – had been sold off, and was used as a restaurant. It became vacant, and was acquired by an aromatherapist, one of the practitioners at Napiers. The old restaurant was converted to consulting rooms, and (at last) a modern toilet for patients. The two basements were knocked into one, and the manufacturing and storage facilities almost doubled in size. It was then possible to begin modernising them, and bringing them up to the standards of efficiency and hygiene demanded by new regulations.

A new branch of Napiers was established in Glasgow, and a second one in Stockbridge, Edinburgh, and both of those were designed and decorated in the distinctive Napiers style. Both were clinics, with several consulting rooms, and since these were designed from scratch, could incorporate all that had been learned over the previous few years in the original premises.

With the new shops, and also with a steadily growing mail order business, restrictions of space again became obvious, but this time in the manufacturing department. Furthermore, it was also clear that the demands of new regulations, particularly those concerning what was called Good Manufacturing Practice, would be difficult to meet in the basement premises at Bristo Place.

So a spanking new manufacturing facility was set up, in an ancient building in Leith. It had previously been, of all things, a meat pie factory, but, now gutted and completely renovated, certainly met all present and prospective demands of hygiene and capacity.

And so it has gone on. The venerable Napiers business of herbalism has been re-vitalised, brought into a new century and a new millennium. Expanded and modernised, it certainly has been, but it is still imbued with the ethics and ethos laid down by

Duncan Napier, his sons and grandson. In the manufactory, Duncan's old favourite Lobelia Cough Syrup is still being prepared, and he would certainly recognise the familiar smell as the Calendula Ointment bubbles on the burner. I suspect, though, that if he visited today, he would raise one of those bushy eyebrows rather quizzically at the stainless steel vats, the white coats and the hair nets.

Those things are required today, and although no-one at Napiers would deny that they are an improvement, they were imposed on the herbal business after the latest government assault in 1986. It does seem that those assaults happen about every twenty years or so, perhaps as each new generation in the medical professions, the pharmaceutical industry and the Ministry of Health come to again regard herbalism and its practitioners as a threat. Like the previous assaults, that latest one was finally repelled by the assembled forces of the profession and an indignant public. However, each assault does nibble away at the right of qualified herbalists to practise as they know best, and to use those herbs they consider best and most effective. The profession can never lower its guard, and must ever be prepared, and it is, for future onslaughts.

Napiers today has the policy of encouraging all of its staff members to study. Several of the herbalists practising there actually began work on the shop floor, and then undertook the arduous distance-learning course from the School of Phytotherapy. Sponsored by Napiers, and doing most of their required clinical training there, they have successfully qualified under what is in essence a form of apprenticeship.

In 2003, thirty-two herbalists practice in the seven Napier Clinics, together with fifty-five practitioners of other disciplines – oesteopathy, aromatherapy, homeopathy, acupuncture, reiki, therapeutic and sports massage, shiatsu, crano-sacral therapy, naturopathy, Alexander technique, nutrition, reflexology, counselling, hypnotherapy, psychotherapy, and food sensitivity testing... and collectively they offer a complete spectrum of ethical complementary healing. Every one of them is fully qualified and fully committed to the very highest professional standards. Between them, they treat an average off almost 4,000 patients each month. In fourteen years, Napiers of Edinburgh, Herbalists, has changed from being a virtually moribund herbal store to its present position as the premier supplier of complementary healing in the country.

Interestingly, and to my mind unfortunately, the herbalists at Napiers are almost all women. There are 36 qualified herbalists in Scotland, and only five of them are men. It does seem that women have reclaimed their ancient position as the healers. Also unfortunately, as any herbalist will confirm, is the fact that most of those many patients are suffering from chronic illnesses, many of them long-standing, many of them having proved resistant to all the medications of allopathic doctors. If only they had appeared earlier in the herbalist's waiting room, perhaps years of pain and discomfort could have been saved, as I can myself testify, remembering my experience with my old friend the duodenal ulcer, and the way in which it was treated so quickly and effectively by my very first experience of herbal medicine.

It is not often realised that the existence of flourishing complementary practices greatly reduces the undoubted pressures on the National Health Service. Without Napiers, for example, an extra 4,000 patients each month would be seeking help and medications from their GPs Instead they are efficiently and effectively dealt with by skilled professional people quite outside the NHS, and at their own expense.

Of course, several major Asian governments – including India and China – recognise the importance of complementary medicine, and have incorporated it in their medical planning. One major Western Government – Canada – has taken positive steps in the same direction, although, as one might expect, the main reason for that is the simple fact that a flourishing complementary medical scene greatly relieves the pressure on their health service and health insurance companies. There, complementary medicine, and especially herbalism, is being incorporated into national health planning, with self regulation and control. Thus the profession will enjoy a security and a certain future, a situation far removed from that in most of Western Europe, including Britain.

Here, the practise of herbalism has been threatened repeatedly by Government activities. It may be that the Government will not, by legislation, again attempt to make the whole practise of herbalism impossible. They have repeatedly been badly burned when that has been tried. Instead, they seem to be attempting a sort of death by a thousand cuts, where new regulations limit what herbs can be used, how they can be used and by whom, how they are prepared and packed, where and how they can be obtained by the public, and what advice can be given on using them. Such regulations, of course, do not require any legislation or public discussion, but are simply imposed from on high. It is a situation which needs to be closely watched, lest those mysterious 'Powers That Be' succeed in doing by stealth what public protests prevent them from doing in full daylight.

The Herbalist's Apprentice

Keren Brynes MNIMH

Before Napiers

IN 1990 I WAS WORKING in a herbal and health food shop called Muirs in Edinburgh, not very far from Napiers, the long-established herbal business. In fact, at that time Napiers and Muirs were run by the same health food company. Both businesses had gone into a sleepy decline, because there hadn't been herbalists practising on the premises for a number of years. The lease for Napiers was to be put on the market and the plan was for the health food company to reduce its overheads and put all its stock and employees into Muirs.

I had been there for about six months at that point and really loved the job. I felt for the first time that my career was on the right track. I had been interested in herbal medicine and nutrition for some years, and decided to try working in the field, so it made sense to me to get a job in a health food shop to learn the ropes a bit more. I was twenty-three at the time, and had left college some two years earlier with, could you believe it, a qualification in Building. My chosen career at 16 had been selected through teenage rebellion rather than a long-term projection into my future. Like most teenagers I guess I lived for the moment. Girls don't do building! Oh, don't they?

My first experience of working in the health field was during my summer holidays from college. We were meant to get placements in a building-related industry if we could. I didn't. I chose to work with elderly people instead, as a holiday relief care assistant. I really enjoyed that, and although I was quite young I contributed a lot to the people I was working with, helped to brighten up their day and really tuned into their needs. I did this for a couple of summers but didn't see it as a long term career prospect.

My interest in herbs and nutrition started around this time. The first herbal book I bought was a small pamphlet about Devil's Claw, describing how it was a fantastic energy tonic as well as helping arthritis and so on. I was sold. I went to my local health food shop and bought my pack of Devil's Claw tea, (which I didn't really need!) and religiously took it until I finished the pack. Then I discovered evening primrose oil, then echinacea and so on. I wasn't just sold, I was definitely hooked and wanted to find out more.

I had been out of college for about a year and a half when the job at Muirs was advertised in the *Edinburgh Evening News*. I applied, got an interview, and was told I didn't get the job. I was so disappointed. Two days later I got a phone call asking me if I was still interested, as the woman who had been offered the position had turned it down. I accepted and started work within a week.

I learned a lot in those first six months, although there was no structured training in place. I felt I was really helping people make a difference to their health. My employers were really pleased with my progress. They should have been; I was a real grafter and quick to learn. It turned out that they weren't the only ones who were appreciating my efforts.

The Early Days

It must have been at the beginning of October 1990 when Dee Atkinson walked into Muirs and deliberately within my earshot said that she was looking for a herbal dispenser. I took this as an invitation to approach her, and popped into her clinic next door to Napiers shop the next day to find out more. It turned out that Dee was taking on the Napiers lease with a view to once more re-establishing Napiers as a household name in herbal medicine, and she invited me to join her. She offered me a proper apprenticeship-style training in herbal medicine, funding a course at the school of herbal medicine in Sussex, while working in the Dispensary making the herbal remedies.

How could I resist? It seemed a like a dream come true. I handed in my notice to the company I was working for, and was pleasantly surprised when they also offered to pay for me to train as a herbalist.

They saw lots of potential for me with their company in the future and tried to talk me out of going to work for Dee. I couldn't be talked out of it though, it felt so absolutely right. My experience is that you should always listen to gut feelings.

By November 1990 I was working with Dee at Napiers. There was a small team of us at first. Dee's parents were there helping. Rene, her mother, was the receptionist for the clinic and Tom her father, was helping in the shop and dispensary. Jacqui Hazzard was the shop manager and Margaret, whose second name I forget, was working in the manufacturing, stirring the lotions and potions. Tom was helping Jacqui in the shop at first, and he became a bit of a celebrity. All the older ladies would come in and ask to speak to him, thinking he was Mr. Napier. Even when it was explained that he wasn't Mr. Napier, they still wanted to talk to him, with the white hair and the Atkinson charm.

When we first got the keys to the premises it was like walking into a time capsule. There were cupboards in the basement that had been untouched for twenty or thirty years. Out came old recipe books, medical equipment, jars of tapeworms and old bottles. It was like a museum down there in the basement. We dusted our treasures down and put them on display in a lovely oak cabinet in the shop, Bob the tapeworm being our star exhibit – 48 feet long, the label said, although we didn't measure him.

Dee at that time had a large number of regular patients and word soon spread that Napiers was the place to go for professional herbal advice. Gone were the days of dusty bags of culinary herbs and cluttered shelves that I remember from my college days. Napiers was once more leading the way with herbal medicine.

Jacqui was in her second year of the herbal course, so I learnt a lot from her, and Dee gave us regular training sessions. The whole concept of Napiers was that people would receive proper advice about herbs and nutritional supplements from trainee medical herbalists. That is a relationship that still works very well, because as a student you can learn so much on the shop floor and the customer benefits from your training.

It wasn't long before Napiers was bustling; word of good service soon spread, and we often had a queue of customers waiting to be served. More staff were needed and taken on, more trainee herbalists were going through their apprenticeship.

In the early days manufacturing was run from one small room downstairs under Margaret's supervision. Margaret had been with Napiers for about twenty years and knew all the old recipes. She was responsible for producing lobelia syrup, pokeroot ointment, blood purifying tonic and so on. We would take turns to help with the manufacturing, tincturing herbs and pouring the ointments so we got a really good understanding of the whole process from start to finish.

At that time my main duties were in the dispensary, making up prescriptions for Dee's patients, and like any good apprentice, sweeping the floor. We all worked really hard, it was a labour of love. The door shut at 5.30 pm, but we were often there much later getting ready for the next day's work, setting up displays, filling shelves and catching up on the dispensing.

When I look back now I'm amazed at how much energy I must have had to work full-time in a busy and sometimes stressful job as well as undertaking a diploma in herbal medicine in my spare time. It's definitely easier when you are twenty-something. It took about ten hours of study each week to complete coursework, but like most students I wasn't always the most disciplined person, and had to sometimes play catch-up if I hadn't been at my desk as much as I should have been. Of course at exam times I studied every hour that I was awake and wasn't on the shop floor working.

Education

The course that I took was with the School of Phytotherapy in Sussex. At that time, this was the only place in Britain you could study herbal medicine. It was correspondence training with an annual seminar down in Sussex at the school. In addition you had to undertake five hundred hours clinical training, either observing a herbalist working, or towards the end of training, taking patients in a supervised setting.

Correspondence work is difficult; if you are tired after a day's work you really have to push yourself to do any studying at night.

When I started the course I really lacked self-discipline, but by the end of it I was really organised and structured in my approach. I guess partly that's what education is all about. In the first year we studied basic anatomy, physiology, philosophy and *materia medica*. First year was pretty easy in terms of workload, but second year was really hard work. That is when we started the more in-depth studies with the medical subjects. At the end of the second year we sat exams. in anatomy, pathology, physiology and *materia medica*. Third and fourth years focussed more on specialities like dermatology, geriatrics, psychiatry, clinical examination techniques, differential diagnosis and therapeutics. At the end of the fourth year we again sat written exams which then qualified us for our final clinical exam, the one that every herbal student dreads.

From second year onwards you start your clinical hours, and that is where I had a real advantage because I had the opportunity to observe Dee practising on a regular basis. She allowed me to sit in with her on her full clinic occasionally, but the majority of my hours in the early days were in the Free Clinic that Dee ran, and still does, for patients on a low income. This was an opportunity to see a large number of patients over a few hours and was excellent training for me. The waiting room was always packed on a Wednesday afternoon. It still is today.

In my third year, Napiers financed a trip for me to do some clinical training in Canada with Dee's sister Chanchal Cabrera. Chanchal is also a herbalist and has a clinic and dispensary in Vancouver. I spent three weeks there, and observed Chanchal in clinic for about sixty hours altogether over that three week period. I also helped in the dispensary there, setting up manufacturing procedures, training staff and setting up a Free Clinic.

In third and fourth years you start taking your own patients to gain essential experience before you are out there on your own practising. Again, working with Napiers set me up so well for this. It's hard for students to get clinical training hours, especially outwith recognised training clinics. Very few herbalists allow students to sit in with them on a one-to-one basis, and when you are at student training clinic you have to share the patients with all the other students, so perhaps you get to take only one or two patients in a whole day. At Napiers during my final year I took the Free Clinic every week with Dee supervising me. I literally got to see hundreds of patients while I was still training. By the time it came to my final clinical exam. I did feel confident in my abilities, although I was still very nervous on the day.

For that final exam., not only do you take a detailed case history, you also need to be able to perform clinical examinations, very much like a GP would do. We learned how to examine the cardiovascular system, the nervous system, the musculoskeletal system, the respiratory system and the abdomen, and those skills were practised regularly. There were other students working at Napiers by the time it came to that part of my training, and we had a second herbalist, Jill Burns, working from Bristo Place. Each week Jill would teach us clinical examination techniques in preparation for our final clinical examination. This all proved to be so invaluable, not just for the exam, but for what I do in my practice every day.

Working on the shop floor also helps you develop good communication skills. I see that with my own students now; when they first begin taking patients, they always seem that much more confident if they work at Napiers, because they get day-to-day contact with people asking for help.

In April 1996 I took my final clinical exam in London. The exam consists of taking a patient's case history and performing clinical examinations in front of a panel of two herbalists and one GP. The panel gives you a grilling about your medical knowledge, your understanding of pharmaceutical drugs, the use of plant-based medicines and so on. It is a daunting experience, but I knew when I walked into that exam room that I knew my stuff, inside out, back to front. I passed.

The Career Ladder

I've had a rather unique career in that as well as my professional herbal training, I've also gained extensive business experience from working at Napiers.

I started on the shop floor as a dispensary and sales assistant, and by the time I qualified as a herbalist I was Development Officer for Napiers, and in the senior management team.

I was promoted to the position of shop manager in about 1992. I was responsible for all the ordering, staff rotas, banking, internal shop displays, windows, promotions and so on. Everything and anything in fact to do with the day-to-day running of the shop. This was challenging for me because I was good friends with all the other members of staff at the time of that promotion, and it's a real art to be friends with people you have to delegate work to. Fortunately there was never any need for discipline because everyone worked really hard, knew their job well and enjoyed being part of a successful team It was also a lot of fun; we were all younger than we are now, and enjoyed going out for drinks and a social get-together, and that really helped to keep the team spirit alive.

At one point I was managing both the shop and manufacturing, but this was short-lived because it was too much work for one person to manage, and the Napiers product range was constantly expanding to meet the demands of both the shop and the mail order customers.

It must have been late 1993 when a second branch of Napiers was set up in Glasgow. My role started to change a little at that point because the increase in shop staff meant we needed to set up a more structured training programme, dispensary procedures and product manuals. In addition, we needed a corporate image. Initially I spent a day a week working on those various projects but it soon became apparent that this was a full-time role.

I taught myself to use a computer, got a desk, and got started on my position as Development Officer. Initially I had a trial period of six months and was told that in order to justify my salary the business turnover would have to increase by X%. We never did review this because it became apparent just how essential this new position was to Napiers ongoing success. I produced a regular Newsletter, dressed the windows and set up the in-store displays in both branches, wrote and delivered a staff training programme, input into product development, design and packaging and so on. This meant that by the time that we were ready to open a second Edinburgh branch all the structures were in place to make this a much easier task. I think it must have been 1995 when Napiers opened its doors at Hamilton Place in Stockbridge.

I continued to work for Napiers in this role until I qualified, at which point I gradually reduced my hours, partly because I was spending more time in clinic, but also because a lot of the job was done. I had set the structures in place and others could continue the work I had started now that they were more experienced. It was time to let other people learn some new skills.

I really value having had the opportunity to work my way up the company ladder and learning the ropes of running a business. So many people graduate as herbalists and have no idea how to set themselves up in practice, how to promote themselves and how to organise their practice as a business. Unlike many herbalists, I have never had any qualms about charging patients or making a profit. One has to make a living from it, just like everyone else makes a living from their chosen career. You can't concentrate on making people better if you sit fretting about the pennies.

In Practice

Once I qualified there was room for me to practise from Napiers Bristo Place branch. I consulted every Monday, Tuesday and every third Saturday, plus I took the free clinic every second Wednesday afternoon. Thursdays and Fridays I spent working for Napiers on my development role, producing the Newsletter, dressing shop windows and training. Gradually over time I passed the administration duties and free clinic on to other up-and-coming herbalists in Napiers, and devoted more time to practising.

I can remember when I first qualified wondering what my next patient would come in with, and hoping I would know how to help them. Ninety-nine percent of the time I did know, but if I did have any doubts I could always turn to Dee for further advice. In those days we did not have an official mentorship scheme with the National Institute of Medical Herbalists, but I had my personal mentor in Dee, who was always there for me, encouraging and supporting me through my training and my early days in practice. I still see patients now who came to see me all those years ago. I have a lady who used to come and see me in the Free Clinic when I was a student; I still see her on a regular basis.

Napiers is the busiest herbal practice in the UK, so in a very short time I had seen a large number of patients and gained valuable experience. I reckon in my first year I saw as many patients as some herbalists see in five. You really get to gain experience very quickly working somewhere like Napiers, and that's why the practice has such a good name because we are all experienced practitioners.

I love what I do. I feel so fortunate to have a job which feels so worthwhile, so valuable and so appreciated by other people. It's hard work being a herbalist, seeing patients all day, being supportive, listening to their troubles, prescribing treatments and so on. Usually the work doesn't stop when you walk out of the door at night. There are often talks to be given, articles to be written, reading to do and of course admin work. Most of the herbalists I know work really hard, but we all need to. It's a growing field, and it needs to be nourished and fed constantly.

What I get from my work is a real sense of achievement and fulfilment. I can't imagine doing anything else for a living. When someone comes back and tells you that you have helped them get better from a problem they have had for a number of years, or when the once infertile couple bring in their new baby for you to see, it feels good with a capital 'G'. Not everyone gets better with herbal medicine. I found this really hard at first; success is always much easier to deal with than failure. But I've learned to live with this because the positives definitely outweigh the negatives. I help a lot of people who haven't been helped by conventional medicine – people from all walks of life with all sorts of problems.

I see a lot of gynaecological complaints, irritable bowel syndrome, fatigue, urinary troubles, stress related illnesses and skin problems. I'll try my hand at treating most problems because there is usually something to be gained by improving one's diet, taking herbal remedies and making lifestyle changes. I have a particular interest in treating skin problems, and run a Skin Clinic for Napiers. I seem to get good results with skin problems, but what I need to do is to start recording this so that I can pass this knowledge on. You start to see patterns with different complaints, and I hope to be able to use the Skin Clinic as a research tool, so that I can pull my knowledge together, and perhaps write a book on the subject, and most certainly run a seminar about skin problems for other herbalists. Plus, most important of all, help people get better.

For me being a herbalist is more than being a practitioner, it's a way of life. Wherever we go in the world we have plants, they are central to all of our lives in some way, they provide us with shelter, with fuel and with medicines. Working with them day-to-day makes me feel connected to what really matters – good, honest, simple living.

I have a herb garden at home which is really important to me, and I try to get out and about during the summer months on herb-spotting walks. I take people out on guided herb walks and try to educate them about the medicinal uses of common indigenous plants. At the moment I still live in Edinburgh and practise two days a week from Napiers, but over the longer term I would like to move northwards to live a more rural existence, grow my own vegetables and live in a more natural way.

That's the real beauty of being a herbalist. I can work almost anywhere there is a reasonable population. I set up my own practice in Kirkcaldy about three years ago and I recently set up a new practice outside Crieff. My plan is that I'll eventually make my living from these two practices and live either in Fife or Perthshire. I would like to have a family, so I need to be able to work part-time and still bring in a reasonable income. This is something I can do as a herbal practitioner.

The only one problem with this plan is that eventually I will have to leave Napiers. I feel like part of the fixtures and fittings there, so leaving that would be a real wrench for me. However, there are other herbalists qualifying every year through Napiers apprenticeship, and I'll make way for someone else to have the opportunities that I have enjoyed.

I've now spent a third of my life working with herbal medicine. I've learned a lot and I know I'm a good herbalist. What excites me is the possibilities that lie ahead and I think about how much I have to learn and how much more I'm going to know in years to come.

I shall be a Wise Woman, and I am a happy woman. What else could one want?

Traditional Herbalism in Scotland

Heaven preserve us from the illness that whisky will not cure.
Old Highland saying

THE SCOTTISH HERBALIST OF today has a very considerable armoury of herbs available to treat illness. Herbs and herbal products are imported from very many countries, and the herbalist is trained to use them, as well the native products of the country. Today, there is a considerable body of knowledge acquired from other countries: for the first time in history, the herbalist is able to utilise the experience and learning of virtually all the non-European systems of healing, as well as the traditional knowledge indigenous to her own country.

In the past, of course, this was not so, and the healer was confined to using only those herbs that grew locally. Moreover, even that was limited by the seasons, since spring-flowering herbs, for example, were not available in the depths of winter and not all herbs are amenable to drying and storing for later use out of their season.

Another factor which affected the use of herbs was changing land use. Plants which flourish under one type of agriculture may virtually disappear, or literally become extinct, under another. We can't even guess what plant wealth is disappearing for ever, as Amazonian forests, for example, are clear-felled for short-term cattle ranching to feed the carnivorous habits of the hamburger eaters. Nor can we know now what plants grew on the vast prairies of the United States before those oceans of grass disappeared under endless fields of grain.

At least in the Highlands of Scotland, we are fortunate in that changes in land use have been slow and few. The ancient forest of Caledonia disappeared long ago, and it is the fairly recent introduction of heavy breeds of sheep which is responsible for the last major changes. And even that took place about two hundred years ago, so that our knowledge of Highland herbs and their use in healing is as relevant today as it would have been two centuries ago.

It must be stressed that healing in Scotland in the past was probably as much faith healing as herbal. The Wise Women, skilful if untutored psychologists as they were, made much use of healing incantations, healing wells, healing threads, healing stones and other devices to encourage the sick to use their innate powers to heal themselves. Even today, little is known, and less is accepted, of the power of the mind to control the physical, in sickness, in health and in the process of healing.

As already noted, we can speak glibly of the placebo effect, where a totally inert substance, handed out confidently by some authoritarian figure such as a doctor, will, in fact, result in healing. We have no idea how it happens, but happen it certainly does. We know that much illness is actually self-limiting, that is, with time, it will go away. (Take the tablets three times a day: your cold will be cured in a week. If you don't take the tablets, it will go away in seven days.) What presumably happens with the placebo is that the mind is tricked into encouraging the body to restore its natural balance of good health, and the healing stone or incantation, used with authority, does just the same. It is a method of treatment used by shamans (scornfully called witch doctors) in virtually every society since time immemorial, and by the psychologists of today.

Of course, such things can work only if the sufferer believes in them, and in the power of the shaman or Wise Woman or doctor.

In preparing this list of herbal remedies historically used in Scotland, and especially in the Highlands, I have noticed how many different herbs were used for treating the same problem. To some extent this must have been due to what grew in different areas, but also to the seasonal availability of the herbs. For the old-time herbalists to have learned all of this implies much experimentation over a very long period of time, and it implies also the careful passing down, generation to generation, of that knowledge. Sadly, that folk knowledge is now dead, and although much has been recorded in recent years, very much more must have been forgotten, and is now lost for ever.

Those folk doctors fortunate enough to have a piece of land were able to grow many of their own herbs. The kitchen garden could stock both the pantry and the medicine cabinet. In the early 19th century the garden of Martha Pollard, a midwife, included turnips, parsnips, peppers, currents, quince and rhubarb, for food as well as medicine, but also anise, burnet, catnip, chamomile, coriander, feverfew, flax, garlic, hops, hyssop, mandrake, marigolds, mint, mustard, parsley, peppermints, rue, saffron, sage, savory, spearmint, tansy and numerous others. Martha Pollard mostly used herbal teas in her cures, for everything from 'stomach colics' to 'sore travel' (travail, or labour).

In the following partial listing of herbs used in Scottish, and particularly Highland, herbalism I have thought it best to use some technical terms. Rather than repeating that such-and-such is used for treating intestinal worms, for example, I have merely noted that it is, for example, a vermifuge or anthelmintic. Those technical terms are:

Alteratives

These herbs act as general stimulants to the body's metabolism, and thus enhance all bodily functions. They stimulate the elimination of waste matter from the tissues. Once known as blood purifiers, they also have a considerable effect on the skin and the digestive system. Bladderwrack seaweed was one alterative herb used in the Highlands, as was red clover.

Amphoretics

These are normalisers, herbs which regulate the body or a bodily organ, and help to restore a state of harmony. Amphoretics act in what seems to be a strange and contradictory fashion, according to the body's own requirements. For example, hawthorn will either raise or lower blood pressure as required. Oats will stimulate or sedate the nervous system according to the needs of the body.

Antihistamines

These herbs, as the term implies, arrest the body's production of histamines, and since it is histamines that cause allergic reactions, antihistamines are used to treat allergies such as hay fever. Elderflower and marigold were perhaps the most commonly used in the Highlands.

Antilithics

Antilithic herbs prevent or cure the formation of stones and gravel in the urinary system, and also help the body to remove them – often painfully. Butterbur was one such herb used in the Highlands. Common cromwell and golden rod were others.

Antiscorbutics

Herbs that relieve or cure scurvy. Almost unknown today, at least in the developed countries, scurvy used to be one of the most common and often fatal diseases. It is caused simply and solely by lack of vitamin C in the diet, and is cured simply by including almost any green stuffs or citrus fruit in the diet.

In the great days of European voyages of discovery and exploration, the greatest enemy was not 'savage' tribes or great storms or unsuspected reefs, but the diet of dried or pickled meats and hard-baked biscuits. The results of that diet was scurvy, when the men's mouths became grossly inflamed, they were totally lethargic, their teeth fell out, the slightest scratch or wound or bruise became infected, and eventually they died in misery. Whole great navies became totally useless and ineffective. Whole army expeditions perished. And all because they were not provided with a modicum of green vegetables. It took literally centuries and uncountable deaths before the lesson was learned, a lesson that any Highland granny could have taught.

Many herbs were used as antiscorbutics in the Highlands. The old custom of the Spring tonic was an opportunity of dosing with vitamin-rich nettles. The common sorrel, groundsel, hemp agrimony, rose root and scurvy grass were all used for the prevention and cure of scurvy.

Antispasmodics

These herbs ease muscle spasms and cramps and over-contractions. That is, they are a muscle relaxant. Since the days of Hippocrates red clover has been used for this purpose, and meadowsweet is another herb widely used in the Highlands.

Antitussives

These herbs reduce the severity of a cough, ease expectoration and clear the lungs. There are very many herbs which have this effect, amongst them coltsfoot, comfrey and thyme.

Astringents

These herbs contain tannins and act to tone up mucous membranes and reduce secretions and discharge. They also help to stop bleeding by forming a scab over a wound. Golden rod, ash tree leaves and bearberry were widely used as astringents in the Highlands.

Bitters

Bitter herbs stimulate the digestive functions and increase the production of digestive juices. Their function is complicated, but very interesting. To be effective, the bitterness of the herb must be tasted. If you disguise the bitterness with a sweetener it will not work. There is a reflex action from the taste buds to the brain, then through the vagus nerve to the gut, where the production of the necessary juices is encouraged, and furthermore the peristaltic action of the intestines is encouraged. It is that peristaltic action which moves the contents of the bowels down, and eventually out. A decoction of ash tree bark was used in the Highlands as a bitter, as was an infusion of feverfew.

Carminatives

These are herbs which relax the digestive system, and promote smooth and regular contractions of the muscles around the gut. They act to ease griping and flatulence. Such herbs are rich in volatile oils, and include mugwort, wild mint and thyme, and these were probably the most used in the Highlands.

Demulcents

These herbs contain a great deal of mucilage and this soothes and protects irritated or inflamed tissues. In doing that, they allow and encourage the natural healing processes to occur. Chickweed is one such, and coltsfoot another.

Diaphoretics

These herbs promote sweating and fever. They act best when the body is already feverish, and thus encourage the body in healing itself. To understand that, one must appreciate that a fever is part of the body's natural defence system. Both bacteria and viruses are most active at normal body temperature, and the immune system is most active at a higher temperature. Thus the diaphoretic herbs, by encouraging the fever, help the body to overcome the invaders. The herbs also help the production of white blood cells, whose task is to trap and destroy the invading bacteria or virus. The sweating is a process of internal cleansing of toxic wastes. Elderflower was used as a gentle diaphoretic and thyme as another.

Diuretics

These herbs promote the flow of urine. They help when there is retention of water in the body, and also help in treating urinary tract infections by flushing out the invading organisms. There are very many diuretic herbs available, but the common dandelion was (and still is) perhaps the most widely used by herbalists. Its country name of 'piss the bed' tells you why, although a herbalist will explain that dandelion contains a great deal of potassium, and that an increased flow of urine depletes the body's essential stock of potassium. Most chemical diuretics must be supplemented with potassium tablets: the simple dandelion does not.

Febrifuges

A febrifuge helps to reduce and shorten a fever. It must have been difficult for the healers of old to decide whether they should encourage or reduce a fever, that is, whether to use a diaphoretic or a febrifuge. After all, it was known that a fever was often part of the healing process, and to reduce it might be harmful. It seems likely that in treating a simple cold or flu, the fever would be encouraged, but it would often be thought advisable to shorten the time of a fever by using herbs which dilate the blood vessels near the skin, and thus allow the internal heat to escape more easily. Elderflowers, thyme and raspberry leaves have this effect.

Laxatives

These are herbs which encourage or promote bowel movements. As there are many herbal diuretics, so there are many herbal laxatives. Perhaps no medication is so widely misused as laxatives, both herbal and chemical. Habitual use of a laxative encourages the bowels to become lazy, as it were, and to depend on the assistance of the laxative. Constipation is best treated, long term, by changing the diet, although the occasional use of a laxative is acceptable. Dandelion root, yellow dock and burdock were common, and gentle, Highland laxatives.

Sedatives

Sedatives calm the body's nervous systems and promote relaxation and possibly sleep. Examples of these calming herbs are primrose, mistletoe and St. John's Wort.

Styptics

Or *Haemostatics*. These are agents that arrest bleeding. They work by helping the blood to coagulate and thus stop blood flow from the wound. Bramble leaves were used for this purpose, as also was St. John's Wort.

Tonics

These herbs increase 'tone' in a tissue or an organ – that is, they encourage the proper functioning of the body or a particular part of it. They act as a mild stimulant. Gowans (Ox-eyed daisy) was used as a general tonic, as was ground ivy. Heather tops act as a lung tonic, and scullcap as a nervine or general nerve tonic. Hawthorn has long been used, and still is, as a cardio-vascular tonic.

Vermifuges

Now properly known as *anthelmintics*, these herbs destroy intestinal worms and expel them from the system. In the past, as now, a herbalist would choose the vermifuge according to the particular worm concerned – male fern (rarely used today) for tape worms, groundsel for threadworms in children and milkwort for adults.

Vulneraries

These are herbs which promote healing. Most of them are astringents, which help to stop bleeding and promote a crust or scab to form over the wound. Common sorrel, hemp agrimony and Herb Robert were frequently used as vulneraries.

Anyone consulting a qualified herbalist today will probably be given a carefully considered and scientifically evaluated prescription of herbal tinctures, tablets, creams or teas. These are all produced in up-to-date, antiseptic conditions, where the required Good Manufacturing Practice is followed, and the medications are standardised.

It was not so in the very recent past, and of course it was not so in the Highlands of yesteryear. The old Highland herbalist used handfuls of the fresh or dried herbs, gathered when experience said they were most potent, and used the simplest of preparations. Generally, she would use a single herb: today the prescription almost certainly contains five or six different herbs, each designed to support and supplement the rest.

The ill person, then as now, would have been instructed how to use the herb, using just the simple methods possible at the family hearth. An *infusion* was perhaps the most used.

An infusion is no more or less than a tea made from a fresh or dried herb. The herb is steeped for a few minutes in boiling water, and then the liquid is allowed to cool a little, strained, and then drunk. This is a very effective way of extracting the medication from the herb, and one still in common use today. However, it only works on the leafy parts of plants, and only extracts those things which dissolve in water.

For roots, seeds and woody stems, it is necessary to make a *decoction*. For this, the plant material is cut or ground or crushed as fine as possible, then simmered, covered, for twenty minutes or so. Neither infusions nor decoctions will keep for more than a day at most, and should be prepared fresh each day.

Fomentations are used externally. They are made by soaking a cloth in a liquid previously prepared either as an infusion or a decoction, and then applied to the ulcer, wound or skin eruptions. Fomentations are usually applied hot, and bound in place with a cloth to keep the heat in. They are renewed every hour or so as long as necessary, or at least until patient or healer runs out of patience.

A *poultice* is the application of the actual herb to an external wound or eruption or to the site of a bruise or fracture. Usually the herb is fresh and green, and is cut up as finely as possible, or pounded, and then applied to the site and bound in place and kept in place for several hours before being replaced.

Ointments were made by simmering the cut or bruised herbs in fat, usually animal lard, for twenty or so minutes, then straining out the herb and letting the resultant ointment cool before applying or storing it as required.

Inunctions do not seem to be used at all these days. I think that method of using herbs must once have been at least known if not widespread, since one of the legends about St. Columba, 1,500 years ago, is that he used an inunction to effect a cure. An inunction is a wad of macerated herb applied to the armpit or groin and bound in place. The healing properties are then absorbed through the particularly sensitive skin of those sites.

The legend of St. Columba does not tell us whether the saint macerated the herb by chewing it. That is the method still used by healers in societies other than our own, where the use of inunctions is still common. I do find it difficult to envisage our herbalists of today busily chewing at a mouthful of fresh herbs then sticking the resultant pulp into the armpit of the patient, and certainly do not anticipate that treatment with inunctions will ever again become popular.

Both infusions and decoctions extract from the herb only those elements which are soluble in water. Long ago, it was discovered that alcohol has the ability to extract those and also other constituents with useful properties. Today, your prescription from a herbalist almost certainly consists of a tincture, which is made by soaking herbs, fresh or dried, in a mixture of water and pure alcohol, and this mixture extracts virtually all the healing properties from the herb. In the past, the Highland healer frequently soaked her herbs in home-distilled whisky, thus producing a rather crude version of what today we call a tincture. There was nothing strange about that, for in those happy far-off days, whisky was not bought, grudgingly, from the local store, but was distilled as a matter of course in every household. It would surely be easier to persuade the sick Highlander to take his medicine in a good dram of whisky than as a pint of herb tea. It would be so then: it would be today.

Herbs commonly used in the Highlands

To use on... wounds and broken arms,
Some had their salves and others worked their charms,
And sage they drank, and likewise remedies
Of herbs, for they would save their limbs with these.

Chaucer

Alder (*Alnus glutinosa*) One of the most common and useful trees. The wood is long-lasting and beautifully grained. As well as being used as medicine, alder produced several dyes from its various parts – red, yellow, cinnamon and green. A tonic and astringent, a decoction of the bark was useful for bathing swellings, particularly of the throat, and was also used as a gargle for sore throats and for external ulcers.

Ash (*Fraxinus excelsior*) Another common and useful tree, with valuable timber. The bark was used as a bitter and an astringent. A decoction of the bark was used in intermittent fevers. The leaves are a diuretic and laxative, being much less griping than other common laxatives. Young leaves, made into a tea, were used for gout and rheumatism, and as a kidney stimulant. Poultices of the leaves were also used for rheumatism. The seed keys were pickled and used as relish. At the birth of a child, the midwife put the end of a green ash stick into the fire and collected the sap which came out of the other end, and gave that as first food to the child. This was believed to be a protection against witches. The leaves give a blue dye.

Barberry (*Berberis vulgaris*) Interestingly, this plant gives a yellow dye, and was used for jaundice. A decoction of the inner bark was used as a tonic, a purgative and antiseptic, being considered particularly useful as a liver stimulant and digestive tonic. It was also used to treat gallstones. It was not used in pregnancy.

Bearberry (*Arctostaphylos uva-ursi*) Records of the use of this plant go back a long way into history. Both the Beatons of the Highlands and their contemporaries the Welsh Physicians of Myddfai noted its usefulness. Only the dried leaves are used. Both astringent and diuretic, it was – and still is – used for toning the urinary system. It was not used in pregnancy or lactation.

Bilberry (*Blaeberry*) (*Vaccinium myrtillus*) The dried leaves were used for diarrhoea. The leaves, infused, were used as an astringent and diuretic, for kidney and bladder problems, and have a strong antiseptic action throughout the urinary tract. The berries are still made into jellies and baked in pies. Long ago, the jelly was mixed with whisky, and given to travellers and strangers. That old Highland custom is, sadly, followed no more. A violet or blue dye was made from the leaves and berries.

Blackcurrant (*Ribes nigrum*) The leaves were used as a diuretic, and an infusion for Spring cleaning of the system. A decoction of the bark was used for stone, dropsy and piles. The juice of the berries was boiled down with sugar and used (it still is) for sore throats, and is both very pleasant and very effective.

Black spleenwort (*Asplenium adiantum-nigrum*) This fern was made into cough syrup with honey, and was also used as a hair wash.

Blackthorn (*Prunus spinosa*) The flowers were used as a laxative, and the berries in fevers and dropsy. A decoction of the bark was used for asthma, and the infused flowers for scabies.

Bogbean (*Menyanthes trifoliata*) This antiscorbutic was simmered and used as a Spring tonic. The stems were decocted for persistent winter coughs.

Bog myrtle (*Myrica gale*) This little plant is a useful insect repellent. Taken internally, it is a vermifuge and a toner for mucous membranes. The roots gave a yellow dye.

Bracken (*Pteridium aqulinum*) This pestiferous plant, which has taken over so much of once productive land in the Highlands, does have some useful qualities. Decoctions of the roots were used to treat intestinal obstructions and spleen problems, and also to treat worms.

Brambles (*Blackberries*) (*Rubus villosus*) Quite apart from the very welcome berries, the roots were decocted, mixed with honey, and used for diarrhoea and dysentery. The juice of the berries is an astringent, and was used as a gargle for sore throats and a wash for mouth ulcers. The young shoots gave a grey dye, and the whole plant an orange.

Burdock (*Arctium lappa*) Alterative, diuretic and diaphoretic, this very useful herb is still widely used by herbalists. It was decocted for use in jaundice and fevers. The bruised leaves were used for ringworm.

Butterbur (*Petasites hybridus*) This strange plant of marshy areas produces its flowers before its leaves, and when the leaves do appear, they are the largest of any plant found in Britain. Those rhubarb-like leaves were used as a useful umbrella. The common name of 'butterbur' refers to the practice of wrapping butter in the leaves during hot weather. A decoction of the root was used as a heart tonic, for inflammation of the urinary tract and for gravel. There are also indications that it was used for whooping cough.

Chickweed (*Stellaria media*) Made into poultices, this herb was used for treating boils and carbuncles. A decoction was used as a slimming aid. Chopped and simmered in fat, the leaves and stems made a good healing ointment.

Clover (*Red Clover*) (*Trifolium pratense*) An alterative and anti-spasmodic, red clover has been used since the days of Hippocrates. An infusion of the flower tops was used against whooping cough and bronchitis. It was also used as a gargle for mouth ulcers and sore throats, with a mouthful being swallowed at each use. An ointment made with flowers simmered in lard was used for eczema.

Coltsfoot. (*Tussilago farfara*) 'Tussilago' means cough dispeller, and it has long been used for that purpose. As long ago as the days of Dioscorides, smoking the leaves was advocated for coughs, and it is still used in herbal tobaccos. Leaves, juice or syrup were all used for coughs, and Coltsfoot Candy used to be popular. Decocted, and mixed with honey or liquorice, the liquid was used for colds and asthma, and a syrup made from the stalks for chronic bronchitis. In Paris, apothecary shops once used coltsfoot as their sign. It is little used nowadays internally, and should not be used in pregnancy or during lactation.

Comfrey (*Knitbone*) (*Symphytum officinale*) A demulcent, poultices were used for healing broken bones and curing wounds. Only used externally today, in days past it was taken internally for lung troubles and quinsy.

Common cromwell (*Lithospermum officinale*) An infusion was used for kidney and bladder stones.

Common sorrel (*Rumex acetosa*) Known as 'gowkemeat' or cuckoo meat, the leaves were infused as a tea used as a diuretic and as a cooling drink in fevers. The juice mixed with vinegar was used against ringworm. The plant was also used as an antiscorbutic and to heal wounds.

Couch grass (*Agropyrum repens*) This is the particular grass, the bane of all those who seek to make a lawn, which is sought out by dogs that are feeling uncomfortable in the stomach. It encourages them to vomit. A decoction of the rhizomes was used as a spring tonic, and also in cystitis. It is a uric acid solvent, and helpful in rheumatism. A plaster was helpful in healing wounds.

Cudweed (*Graphalium uliginosum*) Used for sciatica, an infusion was also used as a gargle in quinsy and for sore throats. A comforting fomentation was used in mumps. The infusion was also used as a hair wash in cases of lice infestation.

Daisy (*Bellis perennis*) The Scots name 'bairnwort' refers to its use in making daisy chains. Do any children do that today? An infusion of the flowers was used as a lotion or compress for sprains and bruises, and an ointment for cuts and bruises.

Dandelion (*Taraxacum officinale*) St. Bride's plant, and Bride was the saint of healing. An effective and well-balanced diuretic, it is also a general urinary tonic. Ulcers were treated with dandelion leaf sandwiches. The juice was believed to heal warts. Roots were dried and used to make a refreshing drink. Dandelion is still the basis for non-caffeine coffees. A brown dye was produced from the roots.

Devils Bit Scabious (*Scabiosa succisa*) The whole herb was collected and dried, then used in scabies. The root was believed to be effective against the plague, and slices held against teeth for quick relief of toothache. The juice of the fresh plant was used for wound healing.

Dogs mercury (*Mercurialis perennis*) Used as a plaster for healing wounds.

Dwarf cornel (*Chamaepericlymenum suecicum*) The so-called gluttony plant. Used to restore appetite after illness.

Elder (*Sambucus nigra*) The Scottish Bour Tree. The bark, which gave a black dye, was a purgative, diuretic and emetic. An ointment of flowers infused in lard was used for wounds and burns. Flowers were used to make elderflower water for clearing freckles, healing sunburn and as a complexion aid to soften and whiten the skin. An infusion of the flowers or berries was used to induce perspiration when suffering from a cold or sore throat. It was particularly effective when mixed with peppermint. Wine was, and still is, made from both flowers and berries. The berry wine in particular, taken hot, induced perspiration, and was helpful for catarrh and sore throats. 'Rob' was very popular. This was made by simmering berries with sugar to the thickness of honey. Taken in hot water at night it was comforting for colds and flu. Most important, in Scotland the tree is believed to be a sure guard against witches, and ideally a rowan was grown at the front of the house and an elder at the back

Feverfew (*Chrysanthemum parthenium*) The fresh leaves, eaten probably with bread, were used for migraine and headaches. The infused leaves were used for fevers and flatulence.

Field Scabious (*Knautia arvensis*) Leaves and flowers were made into an ointment for skin disorders including ulcers, dandruff and even gangrene. It was taken internally for fever, coughs, pleurisy and other lung problems.

Figwort (*Scrophularia nodosa*) Known as the Scrofula Plant. Scrofula, tuberculosis of the skin and glands, particularly of the neck, used to be very widespread. The most popular 'remedy' was to be touched by a king, and the kings of England seemed to have spent much of their time doing that. Charles I is reputed to have touched 100,000 people against the King's Evil, but there is no reliable record of his success. The infusions of figwort used in the Highlands, where kings never appeared, must have been at least as effective as the touch of the royal hand. Poultices of the herb were also used for ulcers, wounds, and generally for skin eruptions.

Flag Iris (*Iris pseudacorus*) This widespread and beautiful flower produces a good yellow dye. The root was powdered and used as snuff for colds, while an infusion was useful in diarrhoea.

Foxglove (*Digitalis purpurea*) The common name has nothing to do with foxes: long ago it was 'folksglove', the glove of the good folk or fairies. It was one of the first plants to be subjected to scientific evaluation in Britain. A Doctor Withering, practising in Shropshire, observed that folk healers in the neighbourhood were having very good results in treating dropsy with infusions of foxglove. Withering himself had little time for botany. In fact, he heartily disliked the botany lectures when he was studying medicine in Edinburgh. However, he became enamoured of a young lady who spent much time in painting pictures of native plants, and in order to engage more closely with her, he began to give more attention to plant life. He knew that dropsy – fluid retention – was usually connected with heart problems, and he observed that the patients treated by local folk healers exhibited a considerable improvement in their heart action. Careful study of the effects of foxglove led him to write a book about it in 1785, and this was a great success. Eventually, foxglove was the subject of close scientific research, which led to the isolation of various glycosides still used by orthodox medical practitioners in treating heart problems. The long use of the herb in folk medicine for heart problems and dropsy was totally vindicated. An ointment made from the leaves was used in treating scrofula.

Gean (*Prunus avium*) The Scottish name for cherry. Tea made from stalks of cherries was used as an astringent, being particularly useful in urinary tract inflammation and cystitis. The gum that exudes from the bark of the tree, dissolved in wine, was used for colds and coughs. A purple dye was produced from the root, and a cream one from the bark.

Goatsbeard (*Tragopogon pratensis*) The bulbous root was a useful vegetable, being used in the same way as parsnips. A decoction of the root was useful in treating gravel and stone, and was also used for stomach troubles.

Golden rod (*Solidago virgaurea*) A yellow dye was made from the whole herb. The flowers are astringent and diuretic, and useful for treating bladder stones. Fomentations of the herb were helpful in healing broken bones. The flower buds gave a yellow dye.

Goose grass (*Sticky willie*) (*Gallium augustifolium*) A tea made from the herb was used as a soporific for sleeplessness and for colds. The herb was also used to make a red dye.

Gowans (*Ox-eyed daisy*) (*Chrysanthemum leucanthemum*) An antispasmodic and general tonic, the gowan was widely used for asthma. The flowers were infused for coughs and bronchial catarrh, and the juice boiled with honey for coughs. It was also used for healing wounds. A decoction of the fresh herb in beer was a treatment for jaundice.

Ground Ivy (*Glechoma hederacea*) Leaves were made into tea and used for consumption and coughs, and a snuff made from the dried leaves for asthma and nervous headaches. It was regarded as being a general tonic, and especially useful for treating kidney disorders. An infusion of the leaves was used for sore eyes.

Groundsel (*Senecio vulgaris*) Another antiscorbutic, this herb was also used as a vermifuge for children. It was also made into a lotion for chapped hands. Boiling water poured over groundsel and thickened with oatmeal was useful for treating festering wounds.

Guelder rose (*Crampbark*) (*Viburnum opulus*) As the common name implies, this was used mainly for cramps and other problems requiring a muscle relaxant. As a nerve sedative and antispasmodic, it was also used for asthma and hysteria. It was also found useful in treating bed-wetting.

Harts Tongue Fern (*Asplenium scolopendrium*) An astringent, this was useful in cases of diarrhoea and dysentery. It was also made into an ointment for haemorrhoids and burns.

Hawthorn or May (*Crataegus oxyacanthoides*) The hawthorn is an invaluable heart tonic, gentler than foxglove, and used in the past when foxglove was not tolerated by the patient, or was not in season. Today, it is generally the herb of choice in heart problems, being a positive heart restorative. It increases blood flow through the heart and strengthens the muscle without increasing the rate of beating or raising blood pressure. The dried flowers, leaves and fruits were all used. The berries were decocted for sore throats, and the flowers and berries made into wine. Children still eat the young shoots as 'bread and cheese'. Leaves were decocted in treating coughs and consumption.

Heather (*Erica and Calluna vulgaris*) The tops of this most common of Scottish plants was a recognised lung tonic and a treatment for consumption and coughs. It is also an anti-arthritic, a diuretic and a nerve tonic.

Hemp Agrimony (*Eupatorium cannabinum*) An alterative and febrifuge, this agrimony was also used as an antiscorbutic. The bruised fresh leaves were used to treat wounds, and a tea made from dried leaves for treating biliousness and influenza.

Herb Robert (*Geranium robertianum*) Infused, the leaves were used for wounds and skin diseases, and a whole plant decoction for digestive bleeding.

Holly (*Ilex aquifolium*) Used for lung problems, the holly leaves were made into poultices for broken bones, and the berries used in dropsy.

Honeysuckle (*Lonicera periclymenum*) Asthma was often treated with a tea of honeysuckle flowers, and the flowers were also made into an ointment for freckles and sunburn. The tea was also useful for headaches. Wine was, and still is, made from the flowers.

Houseleek (*Sempervivum tectorus*) The bruised leaves were used for shingles and burns. The juice was a specific when used on corns and warts, and was wiped over the forehead for migraine. Mixed with warm milk, it was used for fevers.

Ivy (*Hedera helix*) The leaves soaked in vinegar treated corns. Twigs were boiled in butter to ease the discomfort of sunburn. An ointment made from the leaves was effective in treating burns, and a tea for irritated or infected eyes. A bonnet made from leaves sewn together was used for cradle cap in infants. A poultice made from the leaves helped with swollen glands and leg ulcers. For whooping cough, an infusion of the leaves gave relief, and loosened phlegm.

Ivy leafed toadflax (*Linaria vulgaris*) This toadflax gave a yellow dye. It is an astringent, and fomentations made from the fresh leaves are helpful in haemorrhoids. These were also treated with an ointment made from the leaves and lard, and the same ointment used on skin sores and eruptions. A mild liver tonic, the leaves were also used as an antiscorbutic.

Juniper (*Juniperis communis*) The main use made of juniper was in dropsy, when it was often mixed with broom.

Kidney vetch (*Anthyllis vulneria*) A useful ointment for cuts and bruises was made from this vetch.

Lady's Smock (*Cardamine pratensis*) Although helpful in epileptic fits and fevers, little use seems to have been made of this herb.

Male Fern (*Dryopteris filix mas*) Not used in herbal medicine today, an oil extracted from the root of this fern was previously used as a powerful treatment for worms.

Marigold (*Calendula officinalis*) The lovely Scotch Marigold is still, as it was long ago, used in treating skin troubles. Taken internally, it is a stimulant and a diaphoretic, and an infusion of the flowers, or an ointment made from them, is helpful in almost all skin problems. Being a styptic, a tea made from the flowers helps wound healing, although modern practice is not to use it on wounds where the skin is broken.

Meadow Cranesbill (*Geranium pratense*) The cranesbills are an astringent and a vulnerary. They were widely used for healing wounds and external sores. Leaves were pressed against the cavity after tooth extraction, to stop the bleeding.

Meadowsweet (*Queen of the Meadow*) (*Filipendula ulmaria*) This common and beautiful plant had many uses in healing. Like the willow, it contains a chemical very similar to that which was eventually used to produce the common aspirin, and was used to treat the same problems as those for which we use aspirin today. However, it does not have the side effects that the tablets often show. Used as an antacid for digestive problems, it also helps in the treatment of gastric ulcers. An infusion of the leaves and flowers was used for treating colds. As an antispasmodic, it was helpful in treating asthma and whooping cough. Being gently astringent, it was useful in treating diarrhoea in children. In addition to all this, the infusion was used as a wash to keep the complexion clear, and to get rid of skin eruptions. A delightful white wine is still made from the flowers. It was said that lying down, and even sleeping, in a field full of meadowsweet was a certain cure for headaches. The root gave a red dye and the herb a yellow.

Milkwort (*Polygala vulgaris*) As with so many other herbs, the common name indicates its use in healing. Milkwort was used to improve the supply of milk in both cattle and nursing mothers. More than that, though, a decoction of the whole plant was used in fevers. The seeds are a gentle vermifuge, and the powdered root used for pleurisy. It is also a stimulant for the appetite and a regulator of menstruation. It gives a fine green dye.

Mistletoe (*Viscum album*) Very scarce in the Highlands, mistletoe may well have been imported from England for use in healing. Since the days of the Druids, for whom it was a holy plant, mistletoe was used for treating external cancers. The berries are a tranquilliser, and helpful in reducing blood pressure. Perhaps the main use in Scotland was for epilepsy, the dreaded 'Falling Sickness'.

Mugwort (*Artemisia vulgaris*) Used as a spring tonic and appetiser, the common mugwort gave us the old saying:-

> *If they wad drink nettles in March and eat muggins (mugwort) in May,*
> *Sae mony braw maidens wadna gang to clay.*

The plant is rich in minerals, and certainly is an excellent spring tonic, although it should not be used in pregnancy or lactation. It gives a yellow dye.

Nettle (*Urtica dioica*) Long used as a pot herb in spring and as a spring tonic, nettle must be one of the most versatile of all native plants. Fibres were formerly very widely used in weaving instead of flax. In the late 18th century, the poet Thomas Campbell wrote 'In Scotland I have eaten nettles. I have slept on nettle sheets and dined off a nettle tablecloth. The young and tender nettle is an excellent pot herb...I have heard my mother say that she thought nettle cloth more durable than any other species of linen.' The humble nettle, so hated by gardeners and loved by butterflies, was also used as a blood tonic, especially useful in anaemia. It was considered helpful in cases of gravel, and an infusion widely used in chronic diseases. An excellent hair lotion was made from the herb, which also produced a good yellow dye.

Oak (*Quercus robur*) A powerful astringent, oak leaves were used as a styptic. Mouth ulcers were treated with an infusion of the leaves, as were diarrhoea and dysentery. The bark, decocted, was used as a gargle for sore throats. The astringent properties are so powerful that the bark was the most common tanning agent used in making leather.

Orphine (*Sedum telephium*) An ointment made from this stonecrop was used for burns and sores. The leaves, infused in milk, were considered helpful in kidney problems and piles.

Periwinkle (*Vinca major*) Astringent and tonic, an ointment was made from the leaves and lard to heal bruises and piles.

Polypody (*Polypodium vulgare*) The root of this fern is a mild laxative and a tonic in dyspepsia and loss of appetite. A decoction of the root promotes expectoration and was used for treating stubborn coughs. The foliage gives a yellow dye.

Puffball (*Lycoperdon giganteum*) This fairly common fungus was used in treating wounds. Much earlier, in the late Stone Age, there are some indications that it may have been used as a crude anaesthetic.

Primrose (*Primula vulgaris*) The leaves of the primrose are an antispasmodic and sedative, particularly useful in cases of nervous headaches. For treating wounds, the leaves and a suitable fat were made into an ointment.

Purging flax (*Linum catherticum*) This variety of wild flax was infused in whey or water and used as a safe purge, and as a treatment for rheumatism.

Ramsons (*Wild Garlic*) (*Allium ursinum*) The leaves were used as a vegetable, and an infusion as a treatment for scabies and ringworm. A syrup made from the whole plant was very effective against coughs. It was said that 'Garlic and May butter are the remedies for every ill', but then, that is also believed of whisky!

Raspberry (*Rubus idaeus*) Astringent and stimulant, the leaves were used for gargles for sore throats and an infusion for washing wounds. Raspberry leaf tea was a common treatment for conjunctivitis. However, the main use of the raspberry was as an infusion of the leaves to ease confinement. This was, and still is, used in the last months of pregnancy, and during the birth.

Ribwort plantain (*Plantago lanceolata*) Another rich source of minerals, ribwort is an antihistamine and useful for treating hayfever. A decoction of the root was used for fevers and the leaves for wound healing.

Roseroot (*Sedum rosea*) Another antiscorbutic, roseroot was also used in treating skin ulcers of various kinds.

Rowan (*Mountain Ash*) (*Sorbus aucuparia*) The tree was believed to be a guard against warlocks and witches. A rowan tree at the front of the house and an elder at the back was a certain protection. Although it would be difficult today to find anyone who would confess to believing this, nevertheless very many houses, even new ones, are still graced by those two lovely trees planted in the traditional position. Furthermore, making love under a rowan tree was believed to be a certain cure for infertility. More mundanely, a decoction of the bark was used in cases of diarrhoea, and the berries used as an astringent gargle for sore throats and at the other end of the spectrum, as a lotion for piles.

Royal Fern (*Osmunda regalis*) A decoction of the root of this fern was used to treat jaundice, bruises and lumbago. Poultices of the boiled root were used for arthritic joints, and an ointment made from the root for wounds and bruises.

Sage (*Salvia off.*) Widely used to treat sore throats, it was also used – and still is – to treat hot flushes in menopause. It was also said to arrest breast milk production. Furthermore, an old saying attests to its popularity: 'Why should a man die that has sage in his garden?' Also:

> *He that would live for aye,*
> *Must eat sage in May.*

St. John's Wort (*Hypericum perforatum*) For long used in healing, even today St Johns Wort is still one of the most useful herbs in the herbalists' armoury. It was believed to be the favourite of St. Columba, and a legend claims that he was the first to use it. It seems that a young shepherd boy was brought to Columba, suffering from nervousness and afraid to any longer spend long nights alone on the hills guarding his sheep. Columba took a wad of St. Johns Wort, chewed it, and placed it under the armpit of the lad. He was cured of his nervousness, and indeed the herb is used still as a nervine or nerve tonic. It is interesting that the saint placed the herb into the boy's armpit. An inunction, for that is what it was, is a means of getting the power of a medicine into the system without it going through the digestive tract, which might be disturbed by it. The armpit and the groin were used as sites for inunctions, long experience having shown that those were the best sites for the application of the macerated herbs. The method of treatment is hardly used these days. The leaves, infused, were used to heal gangrenous wounds. The flowers were used in hair lotions and in gargles for sore throats. Its main use today is as an anti-viral agent, and as an anti-depressant. The buds gave a deep crimson dye.

Sanicle (*Sanicula europaea*) Used internally and externally as an astringent and a healing agent, the whole herb was usually dried. Its astringent powers were used in treating dysentery, for gum troubles, and as a poultice for varicose veins. An ointment was prepared for use on piles.

Scotch Broom (*Cytisus scoparius*) Broom is surely one of the loveliest of all native plants in Scotland, and the sight of banks of the brilliant yellow flowers one of the most spectacular in late spring. Broom flowers at the same time as gorse comes into full bloom, and the sight of masses of both is a wonderful introduction to the summer months. Gorse can be in flower at any time, and there is always a plant or two in full bloom in every month of the year. Hence the old saying that 'When gorse is in flower, girls are ready for kissing.' The tips of broom shoots and the flowers are a diuretic, and helpful in dropsy and bladder and kidney infections. It is also a stimulating cardiac tonic, but should be avoided by those with high blood pressure.

Scots lovage (*Ligusticum scoticum*) A salad herb and green vegetable, it was used for flatulence and indigestion, as a tonic and aphrodisiac, and for consumption. The roots and rhizomes were the parts used in healing, and were also believed useful in treating worms in cattle.

Scots pine (*Pinus sylvestris*) Although so much of Scotland is today covered with the serried and uninteresting ranks of coniferous trees, the only native conifer is the Scots Pine. There are only a few old Scots Pine woods left, and we are more likely to see only isolated and rather lonely trees. The bark was decocted for use in fevers, and the fresh buds in Spring for scurvy. The resin was made into an ointment for boils and sores. A yellow or brown dye was made from the young cones.

Scullcap (*Scutellaria galericulata*) A nervine or general nerve tonic, Scullcap, like St. John's Wort, was used to treat nervous disorders.

Scurvy grass (*Cochlearia officinalis*) As the name implies, this herb was used not only to cure scurvy, but to prevent it. It has always seemed strange to me that folk medicine successfully utilised so many herbs against scurvy, and had done so for centuries, yet the navy and merchant navy, and even the army, refused to accept this simple treatment and preventative, and for centuries suffered outbreaks of scurvy that killed untold thousands of men, and killed them, moreover, in great distress.

Sea aster (*Aster tripollium*) This was used as a wound dressing.

Seaweeds (various kinds) Seaweeds were one of the staples in the diet of coast-dwelling Highlanders, and, after the Clearances, when the only Highlanders left were banished to the shores and beaches, seaweeds became even more important. They had their healing uses too, and were boiled with milk as a tonic for those run down. Seaweeds are rich in iodine, and although the healers of old could have had no knowledge of that, the seaweeds were traditionally used for treating thyroid problems, and of course iodine is a specific for most thyroid problems.

Selfheal (*Prunella vulgaris*) The herb is a useful astringent for both internal and external use. Laryngitis, sore and relaxed throats, were treated with an infusion used externally, and the infusion taken internally for high blood pressure. An eye wash was made from the fresh juice of the plant mixed with milk, and poultices of the fresh leaves used for wound healing.

Shepherds Purse (*Capsella bursa-pastoris*) The whole plant was dried, and made into a tea used for diarrhoea and for haemorrhages in humans and animals. It was also used for kidney complaints and dropsy. It was not used during pregnancy.

Sneezewort (*Achillea ptarmica*) Dried and used as snuff, the herb had the effect that one would expect from the name. It was a useful snuff for clearing the sinuses when suffering from a cold.

Sorrel (*Rumex acetosa*) A diuretic and anti-scorbutic, the most common herbal use for sorrel was to chew the leaves to clear offensive breath, a use gardeners of today still value. Perhaps more important in the past, it was the most common mordant used in dyeing – immersion of the newly dyed cloth in an infusion of sorrel ensured that the colours remained bright and fresh.

Spleenwort (*Asplenium trichomanes*) Again, the common name tells us what it was mostly used for – disorders of the spleen. Decocted, the root of this fern was used for treating particularly stubborn coughs, and also as a hair wash.

Stonecrop (*Sedum anglicum*) The seeds, boiled, were used for itching and other skin irritations.

Sundew (*Drosera rotundifolia*) This beautiful but increasingly rare plant of marshes and swamps is one of the few insectivorous plants native to Scotland. Being insectivorous, the juice of the sundew is caustic – it has to be to digest the insects on which it lives – and those caustic juices were widely used in treating warts and corns. However the plant is also an expectorant, a soothing demulcent and an antispasmodic. It was widely used for asthma, bronchitis and whooping cough. A red or purple dye was made from the plant.

Sweet Cicely (*Myrrhis ororata*) This herb was used for constipation, for coughs and debility.

Thyme (*Thymus serpyllum*) From the number of different herbs used in treating nervous disorders and weak chests, one rather wonders how the Highlander acquired such a reputation for strength and hardiness! None of the herbs surpassed the common wild thyme for those purposes. Thyme tea was once a very popular beverage, and was believed to prevent nightmares. It was used fresh for whooping cough and for colic.

Toadflax (*Linaria vulgaris*) This herb is a purgative and a diuretic. It was used for jaundice and as a flea killer, and a poultice of the fresh herb as a treatment for piles.

Tormentil (*Potentilla tormentilla*) An infusion of the rhizomes of tormentil was used for dysentery and diarrhoea. As an astringent, an infusion was helpful for sore throats and a strong decoction for piles. Stubborn eruptions on the skin were treated with a strong tea. It is such a powerful astringent that it was also used for tanning.

Vervain (*Verbena officinalis*) A febrifuge, vervain was used to treat pleurisy. As an antispasmodic, it was used for epilepsy and convulsions. The herb promotes milk production in nursing mothers, but was not used during pregnancy.

Violet (*Viola reviniana*) The main use of the little violet was in cosmetics. 'Anoint thy face with goat's milk in which violets have been infused and there is not a young prince on earth who would not be charmed by thy beauty'. It was also used in treating skin diseases, and, boiled in whey, was considered useful in fevers.

Wall rue (*Asplenium ruta-muraria*) An expectorant, wall rue was used to treat coughs and shortness of breath. A blood purifier, it reduced bruises and swellings, and helped with kidney stones and jaundice. A lotion was used for dandruff and falling hair.

Water cress (*Nasturtium officinalis*) Very widely used as an antiscorbutic and a spring tonic, watercress also helped in reducing fevers.

Water dock (*Rumex acquaticus*) Although not used for healing, the Water Dock roots were used for teeth cleaning.

Water lily (*Nymphaea alba*) A decoction of the roots was used to heal boils, and a dark blue or black dye was also made from the roots.

Wild carrot (*Daucus carota*) The boiled roots were used as poultices for ulcers, and the leaves infused in honey for wounds and sores. The seeds are a carminative, and used to treat flatulence or wind. The whole plant is a stone-resolvent, and was used in treating stone and gravel. A decoction of the seeds was used as a contraceptive.

Wild pansy (*Viola odorata*) Used for diarrhoea in children, it was also helpful in epilepsy and asthma. A decoction of the whole herb and flowers was used in treating skin diseases and for improving the complexion.

Wild strawberry (*Fragaria vesca*) The leaves were used for diarrhoea, but, strangely, also as a laxative and diuretic. The leaves and roots, being astringent, were considered helpful in excessive menstruation and bleeding piles. The whole plant helped to arrest milk flow in nursing mothers.

Willow (*Salix alba*) Since the bark of willow is, like meadowsweet, a precursor of what we know as aspirin, it is a useful mild painkiller for fevers and headaches, and as a sedative. It is an anti-rheumatic, and relieves muscular pain.

Woodruff (*Asperula odoratum*) The fresh leaves were used in wound healing. It was used in chest complaints including consumption and to improve milk supply for nursing mothers. An infusion was used in treating varicose veins.

Wood Sage (*Teucrium scorodonia*) Used in poultices for external wounds and sores and as a blood purifier.

Wood sorrel (*Sourie docks, beloved of children*) (*Oxalis acetosa*) The leaves were used as a general blood cleanser. It was also used to encourage appetite, and the juice as a gargle for mouth ulcers.

Woundwort (*Stachys palustris*) Again as the name implies, this herb was used to heal wounds. As a poultice mixed with vinegar it was used for boils and carbuncles.

Yarrow (*Achillea millefolium*) An ointment made from the flowers was used in rheumatism. Tea made from the leaves was drunk for colds and rheumatism, and was also used in consumption.

Many of those herbs used by the old healers have survived into the modern herbal materia medica. However, few these days are grown in Scotland, and virtually none collected by herbalists from the hills and glens. The herbs used by the modern herbalist are most often imported from countries where pollution is not yet such a problem. Fortunately, there are some far-sighted individuals who do grow organic herbs, and I have no doubt that they will flourish, as will all organic farmers and horticulturists.

Finally, one last old Highland saying about health, before it, too, is forgotten:

Fart dry and pish clear,
And you shall last for many a year.

Duncan Napier's Autobiography

THE NAPIER FAMILY OWNS a hand-written manuscript which seems to be the draft of an autobiography by the first Duncan Napier. Sadly, it was never completed, and ends abruptly at a very sad and dramatic moment.

Stoutly bound in boards, and with a quarter leather backing, the book is well worn, but still whole. The pages measure 16cms by 20 cms, and are faintly lined for writing. A stamp on the inside back cover shows it to have been bought from Gardeners of South Bridge Edinburgh, University & Stationery Warehouse, and to have been Number One of the Students' Note Books, price 1/- (One shilling: five pence.)

The handwriting, in ink, on each right hand page, is firm and legible, with almost no crossings-out or changes. Some other hand has added pencilled comments on a few of the facing pages, but these are now illegible.

It is included almost in its entirety as a valuable piece of mid-Victorian social history, and as an invaluable glimpse into the making of a great herbalist and healer.

Strangely, it is written in the third person, referring throughout to 'Duncan', and not to 'I'. Strangely also, the writer never refers openly to the Napier family, but always to 'Mrs... N' and 'Mr. N...' Only once does he slip, and refer to 'Mrs. Napier', his adopted mother, and a very strange, sadistic character she seems to have been.

Some passages of the manuscript have not been included. These are long, rather repetitious descriptions of boyish ploys, tales of strange local characters, and some lengthy dissertations on Duncan's spiritual progress, and especially of his conversion to a rather virulent form of anti-Catholicism. The places where cuts occur are all marked.

From an historical point of view, it is sad that the writer did not include any details of how he used his herbs, so that we are left guessing about his treatment of the various cases he describes. I would dearly like to know, for example, how he treated the young lady whose leg was so ulcerated that doctors in Edinburgh, London, Dublin and Glasgow all insisted that it must be amputated. Duncan affected a cure, and for payment the young lady offered to sit in the window of his shop, exhibit her leg to passers-by, and tell them how she was cured by him. Duncan refused the offer.

Chapter 1

Ejected from Home

ON THE THIRD DAY of February 1831 a boy was born in one of the houses in Braid Street, Edinburgh, whose career was destined to be full of remarkable and striking events.

His mother did not seem to have any affection for the blessing conferred upon her, as, filled with an inhumanity foreign to the nature of women, the babe was wrapped in a bundle of clothes, after being a few hours old and taken from the dwelling, and too with the tacit consent of the father.

After being transferred from one house to another, and kept by kind-hearted neighbours, he was at last adopted into the family of a Mr. and Mrs. N..., who kept a public house at Blackhall, a small clachan lying on the Queensferry Road, a short distance from Edinburgh.

While at Penicuik, some few months afterwards, he was baptised by the minister of the parish, the Rev. Duncan Scott. It was found exceedingly difficult to decide upon a proper name for him, but at last it was finally settled that he should be named after the minister, and accordingly he became Duncan Scott Napier.

The family into which he had been adopted consisted of two girls, and a boy named Robert, besides the husband and wife. As is frequently the case in many homes this lad Robert had a special designation by which he was known. He was called 'The Colonel', and at other times 'The Captain'. Duncan, owing to the colour of his hair, was known as the 'Red-headed Dog', thus shewing in what estimate he was held.

Mr. N... had been married twice, and the children were the offspring of his first marriage. This second wife proved herself a woman of a cruel, hard and savage disposition and the lot of the two girls and Duncan was for many long and weary years harsh in the extreme.

Mr. N... was proprietor as well as occupier of Blackhall Inn. A short period after Duncan's introduction to the family, a place was rented at Morningside to which the family removed, hoping for greater prosperity by a largely increased trade.

Morningside was then a quiet, old-fashioned country village, with no tramway cars running along the roads, nor any sound from locomotives ever falling on the ear.

Duncan was now between four and five years of age, and it is at this period that he begins to recollect events.

His stepmother was always harsh towards him, and as Duncan says himself, 'he was trained up under the most cruel discipline now rarely, if ever, known among any family at the present day'.

From early morning till the shades of evening closed in he was being continually railed upon, and whenever his stepmother, as he called her, was out of the way, then the coarse laughter mingled with oaths from the bar-room would fall upon his ears, instead of winning words and smiles.

Duncan had a very attractive manner at this early age, and the two sisters made him their confidant in all their griefs. They had a childish terror of their harsh stepmother, and on many occasions, while sitting round the kitchen fire, with the warm glow lighting up their anxious faces, they would talk in low whispers over the manner in which their father neglected them, all unconscious that during the conversation Mrs. N... had, animated by a spirit of espionage and jealousy, crept with all a drunkard's cunning behind the door to listen if, by perchance, she could hear her name mentioned. She usually carried a large, heavy walking stick wherever she went, on which to lean for support, owing to a slight weakness in one of her ankles. Ere the startled children could escape she was thrashing them with the stick wherever an opportunity presented itself – on head, shoulders, back or legs, it mattered not, so long as she had the consolation of knowing her blows told on them with effect.

This was a regular occurrence, and they would suffer aches and pains for days in succession. It was no wonder then, that the children dreaded to be left alone when their father visited the city, for he was a partial protection to them while he remained in the house.

Mr. N... was a man of a kindly disposition, one of those well-meaning individuals who would suffer much rather than have any disturbance inside his own dwelling.

The Crown Inn at Morningside was much frequented by carriers who often gave their horses a feed of corn, while having a 'dram' themselves. One of the individuals who called twice a week at the Inn was an elderly man, Andrew Nelson, who was in the employment of Sir George Clerk of Penicuik. Andrew, having taken a fancy to Duncan, obtained permission to take him to Penicuik for three summers in succession, and the lad found those days the brightest that had ever yet dawned upon him.

His first journey to Andrew's residence was truly a memorable one, for he was subjected on the road thither to cruel and unexpected treatment. One Saturday he was placed in the end of the carrier's cart. Barely one half of the journey had been accomplished when darkness set in. Still the horse jogged steadily on, although the driver was sound asleep. Suddenly the cart came to a standstill. Andrew wakened up and began shouting 'Toll! Toll'. In a few minutes the gates were opened to allow the horse and cart to pass on their way. And now a strange event occurred. To quote Duncan's own words: 'Andrew seemed to have fallen asleep in a short time, and again wakened up, but did not seem to know at what end of the cart the horse was walking, for instead of giving, as he intended, the lashing to the horse with his heavy whip, he brought it down, time after time, for many a weary mile upon the face and body of myself, till we arrived at our destination.'

As this was his first journey to the country it was a very sombre look-out for the sunny days near at hand. Duncan well remembers being lifted from the cart into the large kitchen close beside the fire, and also the astonishment of the servants in observing the state of the lad's face.

Besides being marked with the lash it was swollen with the tears caused by his deep heavy sobs. Many were the questionings he underwent, but to all and sundry he gave no reply, until one more fortunate than the others, elicited the awful fact that 'the man who drove the horse had been lickin' him a' the nicht since it got dark.' To compensate for this treatment all the servants took the forlorn lad by turns up in their arms and kissed away the tears of 'The Red-headed Dog'...

Duncan did enjoy those golden summer days, the recollection of which cast a halo over his after life. ...

Andrew Nelson was a godly-disposed man. He had family worship morning and evening. The Nelsons were all regular attendants at the Free Church, and were always the first members of the congregation to arrive, generally before the doors were opened... After church services were over the remainder of the day was spent in the good old way, in reading the Bible aloud, with explanations, singing psalms and praying. The lights were then put out, and the family retired to rest.

In after years Duncan used to speak with rapture of the beautiful surroundings amid which it was his lot to be cast in his juvenile years; the well-kept parks bordered with rhododendrons and shrubs of various kinds; the tall and stately fir trees growing compactly together where, when all was still one would occasionally observe a beautiful deer standing motionless for a space, and then bounding off when the least movement was made by the watcher. Many a morning Duncan would receive a 'piece', a small pitcher or porringer, with a little sugar. With other children, he would go to the woods for a day's enjoyment. Rasps would then be gathered, which when pressed into their dishes and a little sugar added formed a delicious appetiser to the bread brought with them.

In riper years, Duncan, when supplied with raspberry jam, often uttered the words 'Penicuik again!', as they brought afresh to his memory those days filled with sunshine and sweetness.

Mr. and Mrs. N...were not on good terms. They had become more bitter towards each other. Mrs. N... was still lame, but gave Duncan his thrashings as a matter of course. But she trusted him with what she was pleased to term her secrets. Mrs. N... had made up her mind to leave her husband. Before doing so, however, she used every means within her reach of collecting as much money together as possible, taking it from the till unknown to her husband, which was easily done, as he was frequently from home.

One day Duncan was called by Mrs. N... A handkerchief containing coppers and silver was then tied firmly round one of his arms, and with many threats and objurations, he received orders not to loiter or stand still for a single moment until he returned home. 'Run all the way to Whitehouse Toll' a distance of fully a mile and a half from the Inn. 'Offer the parcel you have got tied on your arm to the gatekeeper. Get paper notes in exchange, and tell the toll-man to roll up the notes and fasten the napkin firmly on your arm. Return home the way you went. Do not speak to anyone, nor stand still till you come to me again. Remember!'

Duncan, with the fear of the heavy stick before his eyes literally obeyed his instructions. He ran all the way, backwards and forwards, and arrived panting and breathless at his destination. For many a year he journeyed on the same errand. While Mrs. N... was still going on her downward career, robbing her husband of his money, and drinking whisky to stifle the voice of conscience. Many rolls of notes and gold were thus accumulated, and none knew of the circumstances besides herself, save Duncan, the forlorn lad.

When the supply of whisky was exhausted, Duncan with one of the girls, would be dispatched with a 'greybeard' in a basket, early in the morning, as far as Robertson's a wholesale merchant's in the High Street of Edinburgh, to get it refilled.

[NOTE: A 'greybeard' was an earthenware bottle, with a screw cap, holding between one and five gallons.]

On every occasion they were stopped by the night watchmen, who walked backwards and forwards on their beat, with lanterns lighted, and their long cloaks hanging in tatters from their shoulders. The children were always closely questioned as to where they were going, and on what errand, before being allowed to proceed further.

But those times are past and gone, and the modern 'Peeler' takes the place of the watchmen, and does his duty better than those antiquated worthies who have only left a memory behind them that they once existed.

Chapter 11

Dark Days

AT THIS PERIOD THERE was no such scheme in existence as the Education Act, which compelled parents to send their children to school to be educated. Although Mrs. N... thrashed and ill-treated Duncan without cause, and so frequently made his life as miserable as possible, still she endeavoured to put him in the way of obtaining an elementary education. He was sent for a short period to a school in the village presided over by a female.

The girls during the absence of their teacher had, at the dinner hour, to sweep and tidy up the room so that everything was in proper order when she returned. The boy here made good progress, while entering into all amusements heartily.

After having been taught the very elementary rudiments, he was then sent to a gentleman's school close at hand. Robert N... went with him. And here it was again that the Satanic hatred of his adopted mother once more manifested itself towards him.

Instructions were sent to the master of the school that he was to be very gentle with Robert; no punishments were to be inflicted upon him, while he was not to be tasked with many lessons. Of course to the adopted lad no such leniency was to be given, and one is left in amazement as to the reason why they even took the lad under their roof at all...

Duncan never learned the use of a pen while at this school and many years elapsed before he began his attempts to form letters by writing, so that it can easily be understood when this is stated, that the schooling he received was of a very rudimentary kind indeed...

At this period criminals were executed where the crime was committed, or as close to it as possible. Duncan remembers of two men who were taken outside Morningside to be executed. After the law had been fulfilled, they were taken down, having been suspended the usual time. While the cart, containing the bodies, was passing along the roughly made road, one of the men gave signs of life, and soon sat up. Refreshments were then given him, and sitting dejected in the conveyance he was taken back to Edinburgh, there to be dealt with by the authorities.

[NOTE: It is interesting that this recollection of Duncan's is very similar to one of the legends that have accumulated round the notorious Deacon Brodie of Edinburgh, well-known cabinet maker, and better-known house-breaker. Brodie, with his long and successful career as both thief and highly respected member of society, was the inspiration for Robert Louis Stevenson's *Dr. Jekyll and Mr Hyde*. The legend is that, the night before his execution, one of Brodie's mistresses arranged for a doctor to insert a silver tube into Brodie's windpipe, hoping that this would allow him to survive the hanging. After the hanging, Brodie was cut from the rope as quickly as possible, and then he was galloped in a cart over the roughly cobbled streets in the vain hope that this would revive him.

It failed, and Brodie had gone for good, except, of course to be immortalised as Dr. Jekyll, like Brodie, the very epitome of a man leading a double life. It is certainly possible that RLS, writing Dr. Jekyll and Mr. Hyde in 1886, knew of the strange case of the resurrection of the hanged man of Morningside.]

While such events as these were taking place, Duncan's life was not becoming any more cheerful or happy. Mrs. N..., while robbing her husband, made the two girls and Duncan work very hard.

They were sent out to glean in the fields, and had to accomplish a certain amount of work before daring to return home.

[NOTE: To 'glean' was to go out into the fields after the harvesters had finished their work, and pick up the stalks and grain heads inevitably left behind. This was one of the few perquisites available to farm workers and their families in those days, and Mrs. N... must have had some special arrangement to allow her family to do it.]

The girls had thirty bundles to bring back, and Duncan twenty. They received, before starting, a quantity of string, cut into the requisite size – fifteen inches – which was to be tightly tied round the gleaned corn.

Starting early in the morning, wet or dry, each furnished with half a slice of bread, to last them till five, and sometimes eight o'clock in the evening, they were hardly dealt with indeed. Many a night, too, on coming home worn out and weary with gleaning underneath the rays of the hot sun, or cold and wet with the drizzling rain, and literally starving with hunger, they would, instead of a supper receive a flogging and be sent to bed, glad to receive next morning the cold 'brose' or porridge, kept from the previous evening.

Such treatment as this prevented Duncan's proper development, and it is much to the credit of the two girls and Duncan that they never thought of stealing a single article to satisfy their cravings of hunger, although they had abundant opportunities. And it must be kept in mind that Robert did as he liked, and was exempted from all such tyrannical tasks.

Affairs had never prospered with the N...s at the Crown Inn. Mr. N... was always hard up and poverty stricken, yet all the time his wife continued amassing money. Every few days Duncan was despatched from Coltbridge to Whitehorse Toll, running all the way both going and coming, to get the money changed. Here, at Coltbridge the two girls were sent out to labour in the fields, for which they received from their employer twopence each, per day.

Duncan, who had a natural taste for gardening, now began to cultivate a patch of his own, in which he reared cabbages, radishes, lettuces, potatoes, strawberries and other fruits, which he conveyed to the market at Edinburgh in a wheelbarrow, and then delivered up the money received for his produce to Mrs. N... On every occasion she gave him back a penny, which, with other coins received from the neighbours, were carefully put in his 'penny pig' to assist in purchasing clothes for him at a future period...

Meanwhile Mrs. N...'s health grew much worse. Her temper became daily more irritable, while she kept wreaking her vengeance on Duncan and the girls in the usual manner...

Mrs. N...'s usual kind of liquor was 'half and half', consisting of half a glassful of whisky, and then filled to the brim with 'Dick's Small Beer'. When in bed, and she was often lying down now, Duncan was always sent downstairs for the mixture, almost every half hour, generally eighteen to twenty times a day. To this compound, on several occasions, was added a tumblerful of unreduced whisky. Mrs. N... did not drink this off, it is true, at a single draught, but by degrees, so one can have a faint idea of the state of body produced by such awful excesses, and how every womanly feeling would be stamped out of her by such a dangerous habit...

She often made Duncan stand at the door to prevent any person from entering her room, while she was counting over and over again her hoarded money. A servant, Mary B... by name was engaged to assist Mrs. N..., and to lift her in and out of bed...

When Mrs. N...obtained this servant, she had the money, which was firmly tied in a large white napkin, kept beside her in the bed. On one occasion the packet fell on the floor with a dull crash. Mary was very anxious to know what was in the parcel, but Duncan hurriedly picked it up and handed it to Mrs. N... who said 'That's a secret!'

As the lad said himself: 'For many long years afterwards, whenever I heard of anyone having a 'secret', I would think they are well off having one, as of course I imagined a 'secret' meant a large sum of money, such as Mrs. N... had dropped on the floor that day.'

On many an occasion, when in a more genial mood than her usual wont, Mrs. N... would say to him: 'Oh, Duncan! I wish you had been a lassie instead of a boy.' No wonder she said this, for he did a girl's duties around the room, even to giving her the needed medicine. Not withstanding the lad's kindness, however, when she became too weak to lift a stick or the tawse to Duncan, she always gave him to understand that his floggings were only deferred, and that a double one was in store for him, when her health improved, so that a continual sense of impending calamities was always hanging over the horizon of the lad's mind.

Chapter III

Misfortunes and Adventures

MRS. N...'S SAD AND USELESS career was now drawing to a close. As the days glided past she still had hopes of recovery, while keeping count of the number of floggings Duncan was to receive when she was able to move about once more.

Duncan began to calculate on the future, and imagined that Mrs. N... might be kept in bed, and his floggings still further deferred, if she obtained less whisky, so, instead of giving her 'half and half', he gave her gradually more of the beer and less of the stimulant, under the impression that she would not rise from bed so soon.

At this time Duncan was her sole confidant with regard to the 'secret', and he distinctly remembers the occasion when he handed her the money for the last time, when she was unable to rise out of bed herself for it. The day afterwards a Mrs. K..., a washerwoman residing at Corstorphine, was sent for to help Mrs. N... and to do any necessary work. She now received two spoonfuls of wine frequently, and her husband was, in the daytime, in constant attendance at her bedside. All that evening Mrs. K... attended to the dying woman, and in the morning obtained permission to go home to Corstorphine to 'make her husband's breakfast'.

She came back in two hours and found Mrs. N... still unconscious. Duncan was outside flying his kite, but heard from the neighbours that Mrs. N... 'was fast passing on', and at four o'clock in the afternoon she passed away.

Duncan, when he heard of the event, was not grieved. One thought was uppermost. His floggings were past, and that was sufficient for him. When he went into Mrs. N...'s room the bed was empty. Her body was laid in another apartment, but all the time, both before and after the funeral, there was a great stir and bustle constantly going on. Drawers were emptied, receptacles ransacked, papers strewed the floor, and everything was in general confusion. Duncan knew the people were searching for something, but did not understand, till years afterwards, that the 'secret' was the object of their search.

Mrs. N... was interred in Corstorphine churchyard, without her body clothes being taken off, a large white sheet simply rolled round her. Mr. N... now came to believe that the 'secret' had been interred with her. Firmly persuaded with this idea, he resolved to have the body exhumed.

The necessary permission was then obtained. A rumour of Mr. N...'s proceedings having leaked out, a large number of people assembled in the churchyard, and began to throw stones and other missiles at the man who dared do such a deed.

The gravediggers completed their gruesome task, but as no 'secret' was found, after searching, Mr. N... had no reward for his pains, and had heavy expenses to pay. More mortification still awaited him. He had not long returned home when he was handed a bill for payment on account of his wife from an individual residing at Greenside Place, Edinburgh. Mr. N... was quite taken aback at this, and several years passed ere he was able to complete payment of the sum demanded.

Mrs. K... was in very indigent circumstance before Mrs. N...'s decease. Her husband was employed as a cab driver. Not long afterwards he became proprietor of a coach and pair of horses, although having lived in the utmost penury up till this period. Money wrongly come by takes to itself wings, and the after career of the K...s was a short, if brilliant one. It is needless to trace too minutely their career, beyond stating in Duncan's own words the following facts: 'The last time that I saw Mrs. K... and her husband was one day walking across the Grassmarket in Edinburgh in a most deplorable state. She was leading her husband by the arm, and he was carrying a load of shavings tied in a ragged sheet. Oh! What a miserable appearance they presented. They were both bare-footed, and such clothing as they had on their bodies was besmeared with filth, and all ragged and tattered. They were the most miserable couple I ever remember having seen walking the streets of Edinburgh. Mr. N... never saw or heard any more of what was once his own, but remained poor for a long period.'

Duncan, after working for months with a practical gardener, where he was in his element, then engaged himself to Adam Dunn, a farmer. He was now fourteen years of age, and it was at this period, in 1845, that the terrible potato blight made its presence felt over a wide area.

[NOTE: This is the only reference Duncan makes in his manuscript to matters outside Edinburgh. Although not so well known as the Potato Famine in Ireland, Scotland also suffered badly from the blight (*Phytophthora infestans*).

By the late 18th century, population pressure and a shortage of arable land created an almost total dependence on 'tatties' for food in the agricultural districts of Scotland, both Highlands and Lowlands, but especially so in the Highlands. Much of the good arable land had been taken out of cultivation there during the Clearances, when peasant farmers were ejected from their holdings by the landowners to make way for sheep farms.

When the blight appeared, it was catastrophic. Overnight the crops wilted in the ground and the potatoes rotted, with a nauseating stench.

Unlike the situation in Ireland, where many thousands died (perhaps as many as a million or a million and a half people, but no-one was counting), the Government in London acted with sufficient vigour to avoid a collapse of the population. After all, the Scots were needed as reliable and valiant cannon fodder, even if, as General Wolfe cynically wrote before he sent the Highlanders off to storm the Heights of Abraham, and secure Canada for Britain, 'it were not great mischief if they fall'.

Actual deaths from starvation in Scotland were comparatively few, perhaps largely because of the activity of a Government Commissioner, the wonderfully named Sir Edward Pine Coffin. He brought with him two naval frigates to act as floating meal depots, and helped establish a well-endowed Fund for the Relief of the Destitute Inhabitants of the Highlands.

By a combination of persuasion and arm-twisting, Coffin arranged that many landowners supported their tenants with hand-outs of meal. But Victorian charity was not for the undeserving or the idle. In return for a hard day's work on road building, the reward was a handful of meal. Many 'Destitution Roads' were built through the Highlands at this time, by men and women slaving quite literally for enough food to keep the family alive for another day, and we travel those roads to this day. Many of the jetties in the Highlands were built then, and they, like the roads, were of great benefit to the landowners. We stand on those jetties today, and wonder how human hands ever cut, carried and placed those great stones. It was all done by men and women in desperation.

Before relief of any kind arrived, the peasants survived – barely – on what they could scavenge from the sea or the shore. The cattle had gone, the seed corn eaten, and the people desperately malnourished and disease-ridden.

Even the usually docile Highlanders, accustomed to obey their chiefs and the bidding of the ministers, rioted in despair when shiploads of cattle and wagons of grain, belonging of course to the landowners, were exported, while they and their families literally starved. Naval ships and army regiments were needed to ensure that trade was not interrupted.

The blight, and the famine lasted until the 1850s, and the destitution only finally relieved by another wave of clearances.]

... Duncan now got his choice whether he would become a blacksmith or a baker, and chose the latter, when he was then apprenticed in 1846 to Mr. B... in Coltbridge, where he obtained as wages, three pounds per annum and a pair of shoes.
... The present Mrs. N...

[NOTE: It appears that Mr. N... had quickly married again.[

began to try to gain Duncan's friendship, with one end in view of course, and made him a present of pigeons, whose broods he sold at good prices.

She also gave him Russian rabbits, which bred at a good rate, and had often more than forty at a time. He drove a good trade with them, but all the money thus gained was handed over to Mrs. N..., and Duncan after a short period of happiness with his pets having had his beautiful pigeons stolen during the night, and his rabbits maliciously and heartlessly poisoned gave up keeping pets for a long period. Before the catastrophe occurred he had been extremely annoyed with rats, and he found a way of terminating them by mixing dry lime and half-burnt oatmeal in equal parts, and laying beside this a dish of water.

The evil habits of Duncan were now about to receive a check.

[NOTE: It is hard to know what those 'evil' habits could have been. He only reports childish pranks and escapades.]

Up till this period when he was sixteen years of age, he had never tasted water as a beverage. While going with his rolls one morning, he met in with a gentleman to whom he owes his rescue from the thraldom of drink. This was Mr. John Hope, of 31 Moray Place, Edinburgh, whose name will go down to posterity as a man who did good to lead young men and women towards a higher and better life.

After enquiring Duncan's name, the conversation gradually grew more personal and interesting.

'What does your folk do.'

'Oh! They sell drink.'

'What! Sell drink! And do you take any?'

'Oh! Yes!'

'What sort of taste has it got?'

'Very nasty, sir.'

And then Duncan's questioner found that Duncan was unacquainted with water, as yet. For many mornings, Mr. Hope, who used to take an early walk in the direction of Ravelstone House, argued and pleaded with Duncan to give up the accursed drink. But Duncan was stubborn, and did not like the prospect of drinking nothing stronger than cold water.

'Dick's Small Beer' had still an attraction for him, and it was

only when more earnestly pleaded with, and shewn that no drunkard could enter heaven, that he relented and consented to give water
a trial for one month, and there, on the highway, the earnest enthusiast of temperance prayed for God's heavenly help to aid the lad in
his resolution. Duncan was awed at the fervency of the man, and at
the extraordinary interest he took in him, poor and uneducated.

Duncan stood the test successfully, and became a pledged
member of the British League in May 1846, and from that period
never tasted alcoholic liquors, or used tobacco.

... He had to deliver rolls at a public house every morning, and
the landlady used every means to induce him to take a 'nip', but
in vain. She finally gave up pressing him to drink, and was afterwards very kind to Duncan and gave him, on many a morning, a
cup of hot tea and a roll. Her husband, an elder in one of the
Edinburgh churches, was much addicted to drink. Catching cold
while in one of his fits of debauchery, he died in a few days afterwards the death of a drunkard! ...

Duncan now joined one of Mr. Hope's evening classes held at
Tollcross, and walked from Coltbridge every evening to it, a distance
of several miles. He had only received the rudiments of an education
hitherto, and up till this period could not write a single letter, so his
master 'set' his copy, and Duncan began to make the familiar 'whips'
in ink, and gradually grew more familiar with the pen...

In regard to Duncan's Sabbath evenings and how they were
spent at this period at Coltbridge, let us quote his own words: 'I
remember about this period of my life, that along with several others about my own age we met together in a widow's house, who
had two sons, Andrew and James. The latter, who was a good
reader, read the Bible, usually those chapters about Moses and the
plagues of Egypt, each of us asking any questions, and also criti-
cising the part read, which proved very profitable. In this dwelling,
however, there was a very mixed company. There was a large sow,
some thirty stone in weight, with occasionally a litter of twelve
pigs running about the floor, a large number of hens, as well as
rabbits and pigeons' ...

His master, a Mr. B... also kept the Post Office and Duncan for
a year delivered the letters in the outlying districts. He did well at

Christmas time, receiving many sums of money as his 'hansel', from a guinea downwards, so that he had never been so rich in all his life.

Mr. N... seemed to have been a man of a very pliable and weak nature, and the present Mrs. N... had come to the house bringing a daughter with her, aged eighteen years. Her disposition was not one whit better than that of his former wife, as she had a terrible temper. She beat Duncan, big as he was, several times, and the lad, sick at her, resolved to leave the house for ever, although where he would go for a home, he knew not.

Duncan carried his plan into execution, and slept that evening in a haystack, but being found by Mr. N... who had come, with others, to search for him in the morning, he was taken home and received another scolding from his stepmother.

She also thrashed the two girls, and this conduct so maddened them that affairs were soon brought to a crisis. Mrs. N... attempted to beat the eldest of the two girls, and the younger one, driven frantic at so much harsh treatment, rushed to the fireside, and seizing the poker, brandished it excitedly above her head, while she exclaimed 'If you don't leave go of my sister I'll smash your skull!' This threat was sufficient and from this period no more thrashings were bestowed on the sisters or Duncan, although their home life was truly miserable.

When the new bridge at Coltbridge was completed, there was quite a feast of jollity, all the workmen who had been engaged in its erection receiving a fourpenny pie, and so great a quantity of liquor that the people of the neighbourhood came in for a good share, with the result that many scenes of debauchery ensued.

Duncan's mind, at this period, began to be troubled with higher thoughts, and he wanted to become a Christian, so as to be enabled to resist the many snares around him, and fortunately for his future Mr. Hope's teachings came as beacons to light him on his way.

The bakers' hours were at this epoch, generally speaking from three o'clock in the morning till six in the evening, but Duncan frequently wrought on till ten, when he would just be fit to go to bed. Frequently, when going with the rolls in the summer mornings, while walking along the road, he would fall into a sound sleep with the result that his foot, catching in a rut, rolls and lad would be landed together in a heap.

Later, while driving his master's pony, the same thing happened, and many a time he was awakened from his slumbers by hearing a loud 'Hallo!', but he always escaped a collision, although he had many narrow escapes.

A brother of Mr. B...'s having come to spend a few days frequently sat beside Duncan on the van as he went his rounds, and was so delighted with the young man's kindness to the pony (he never used a whip) that two weeks after his return to London, where he had his place of business, he sent Duncan a suit of clothes which were valued very highly. So much was this the case that he was afraid to put them on, but a brother of Mr. B...'s wife persuaded him to 'hansel' them by going to Dr. Guthrie's church with them on, as he had never been inside such an edifice since the day he carried the late Mrs. Napier's stool to the one at Morningside. (NOTE: This is the only occasion in the manuscript that Duncan writes 'Mrs. Napier' and not Mrs. N... One has to wonder why he chose to obscure the name in that very transparent way.)

Duncan consented, and went. He enjoyed the sermon very much indeed, more especially the short stories used to illustrate his subject. He went regularly for a year and a half, and then resolved to become a member of Free St. John's.

... After attending Free St. John's for two years, he was enrolled by Dr. Guthrie as a member, although Duncan was sorely disappointed that the reverend gentleman did not ask him any questions regarding his belief, for Duncan knew although he was a member of a church, he was not converted, and he had to grope in darkness for some years longer. But Duncan tried to do what was right, and never went to bed without commending his soul to his Maker ...

As Duncan says himself: 'Those days were days of slavery to the bakers, as they had to board with the master, and commence work whenever the sponges were ready, which was frequently at two o'clock, and never later than three, and they worked on till six at night.'

Duncan remembers the agitation of the bakers to be put upon the same footing as other tradesmen from five to five, in which the men were successful after an arduous conflict. The weekly pay of the bakers, before this struggle was brought to an end, was from five to eight shillings a week, with their board, so one can understand how difficult it must have been to keep a wife and family in anything like comfort. Besides their pay, they received from two to four loaves a week free.

Chapter IV

MR. N... FINDING IT was useless for him to remain any longer in Coltbridge, removed to the West Port, Edinburgh. The house which he occupied has been demolished, and on its site a Free Church – the Rev. J. Jolly's – has been erected. Duncan, at this period, had been six years with his master. Every Saturday afternoon he went home and stayed till next evening. During this visit he gave his assistance in the Public House by serving customers and doing any necessary work, completely forgetting for the time that he was infringing his pledge as a member of the British League, although he never tasted alcoholic drink.

Duncan was now sixteen years of age. While running off a barrel of ale into bottles in the cellar, he was joined by a young man, a relative of the N... family who asked him why he did not go and see his mother at her shop?

This was an anxious moment for Duncan, and on making enquiries he found that his mother was indeed alive, although he had, as yet, never seen her face.

Shortly after nine o'clock, Duncan went to his mother's shop, and gazed long and earnestly inside. As Duncan says himself: 'One must imagine, for I cannot describe, the strange sensations which flitted though my frame. I stood and wondered, and wondered again, at the past life of sorrow and suffering, and I thought how frequently I had passed and re-passed my mother's door without knowing it. I thought her face and hair was very like my own. I could not venture inside for some time, but at last I did so, and asked for a pound of apples. I began stroking a large cat on the counter, for the sole purpose of attracting my mother's attention, and hearing her voice, in which I succeeded.

'I would have liked to have revealed myself, but did not do so. I made many calls at the shop for about three years, for I could not stay long away, and my feelings were far more curious than I can describe in having found out my real mother.'

Duncan while serving customers in the drink shop at the West Port, saw many phases of humanity. Many of them were of the lowest caste of society, who would have sold their souls for drink, indeed multitudes did so every day......

Duncan's experience of a publican's business was such that his life was sickened with the awful effects he saw the drink produce and the great sacrifices which people made to obtain it.

'The number of licensed shops in the West Port was twenty, and taking the drink sold in Mr. N...'s place as an average, the business done must have been very great. Our premises had a back door opening into a court in which lived vast numbers of the poorer classes who kept themselves always on the verge of poverty by spending their money in drink.

'At the time of which I speak, the Forbes MacKenzie Act was not in operation.

[NOTE: This Act of Parliament, passed in 1853, was an attempt to limit drinking by the working class. Public houses had to close at 11 pm, and remain closed on Sundays. However, *bona fide* travellers were allowed to drink in public houses on the Sabbath, and those determined to drink wore out their shoe leather in trudging the requisite three miles before entering the bars and signing the book declaring that they were indeed travellers.]

We opened our premises as usual, on the Sabbath, at six o'clock, and the only breathing time we enjoyed, as stated in the license, was when we 'shut during divine service'.

'Every morning there would be a number of persons waiting till the doors opened. Some of these had neither a covering on their heads, nor yet to their feet, while the clothes they wore only served to screen their nakedness. Several of these people came with strange dishes for their liquor. One woman would have a large water can, in which she would put half a gill of whisky, and after reaching the well would let a small quantity of water run in, and then raising her pitcher to her mouth, would drink it off in the face of her unsuspecting neighbours.

'Some would have a cream jug on their way to the dairy, and others cups, and so the secret and open drinking went on.

'The old couple were not able to help us on the Sabbath, as they were sleeping off the effects of their debauchery in bed, while four of us were moving to and fro as busily as we could, serving the constant, never-ending stream of degraded natures.

'Others would sit in the boxes and drink till their brains became intoxicated with the effects of the alcohol. They would then become dangerous to their neighbours. Oh! The awful cursing, swearing and yelling within the shop, while out of doors, mobs of people were gathered round those of their number who were fighting, and the shouts of 'Murder!' and the fierce threats and cries which came from infuriated throats made one think of Pandemonium itself let loose.

'Such scenes were not confined to the West Port alone, but throughout the whole of the poorer districts of the city such as the Cowgate, Grassmarket, High Street, Canongate and other places where the fruits of the drink traffic made the Sabbath day hideous.

'As one who knows somewhat of the doing of this traffic in Edinburgh, I have been much astonished at some men who maintain, at the present-day, that the drinking is now as bad on the Sabbath as it was before the Forbes MacKenzie Act came into operation in Scotland.

'I may here state a few facts which will shew to what extent the drink traffic was then carried on. Whisky was sold by us at three pence per gill, and a penny extra had to be paid by the customer if he sat down to drink it. I was always the one who took charge of the drawings on the Sabbath. From six a.m. till eleven, the average drawings were £16; from one o'clock till two £4; and from four till eleven £8, making a total for the day of £28! It can thus be seen that if our business drew so much, and with twenty other shops in the near vicinity doing an equally good, if not better, trade, one can have a faint idea of the awful misery produced to those who patronised such shops, not to speak of the other evils which attended on the drink traffic – but the poor deluded creatures are much to be pitied.

'When the Forbes MacKenzie Act came into operation such

things became almost effete. This Act has been an inestimable boon to Scotland, and although a few unlicensed houses or she-beens have sprung up, this cannot be wondered at, owing to the craving for drink on the one hand, and the loss to the trade, by the stoppage of the traffic on the other. The law officials were not always heartily interested in the putting down of these shebeens. Three of these individuals once said to myself that they would take in hand to put down these shebeens, not only in Edinburgh, but in Leith also, and that in a very few weeks, but they thoroughly believed as long as certain bribes were given, so long would they connive at the traffic, and keep it alive. These are facts which I can prove, ugly as they appear...

'I had to assist in bottling, and also in pumping the whisky out of the casks. Publicans maintain that the person who stands beside the cask and pumps out the whisky must first take a drop himself, or otherwise he will fail in doing his work, owing to the fumes which rise and cause the brain to become stupefied. Of course, when I was set to this kind of work, I was strongly persuaded to take a 'nip', but I just thought that those who gave such advice liked whisky themselves, and it was for this reason that they kept up such a custom, so I said that if I was to taste the drink, I would do none of the work, and they reluctantly let me have my own way with the result that the pumping did not inconvenience me in any way.

'I was often troubled and uneasy when I reflected on the evil that I was assisting in spreading, but this sad work at the West Port was brought to a conclusion in the following manner.

'Mrs. N... accused me, before a number of customers one day of stealing a half sovereign which she found in my pocket. I denied the charge, and stated that I had received it from a Mrs. P... at Coltbridge as my 'New Year', along with several other smaller sums of money from various of my master's customers. Still she would not believe my statement, but began scolding the more. Fortunately, I was cleared from this most unjust charge by the gardener of the lady coming in who stated, after the charge against me had been explained, that it was he who handed me the money, as well as a slice of short-bread, and that he knew I had always obtained the same since ever he went to Coltbridge, which was the truth.

'When all was over, however, and my innocence established, I was so overcome that I cried bitterly, and after a few minutes, I said to all those present 'From this night I will never more sell, nor handle, drink, nor even walk behind the counter of their shop again, since I have been accused so falsely.'

'And I kept my word.'

Mr. N...'s business had now increased to such proportions that the landlord intimated his intention of adding twenty pounds a year additional rent. Mr. N... would not consent to pay such an exorbitant price, so he looked about for other premises, which he found in Abbey Strand, where he opened a place under the name of the Crown Tavern. Here, on the Saturday evenings, to draw custom, a Free and Easy was instituted, which was chiefly patronised by glass blowers and carters. Duncan still continued to spend his Saturday evenings in town.

Duncan says: 'I remember visiting one of the Free and Easy's in the Canongate. The apartment was filled with a haze of tobacco smoke. At the far end of the room a stage was erected on which two men with blackened hands and faces were reciting and singing to the amusement of their auditors.

[NOTE: This is an interesting statement. The entertainers had 'blackened hands and faces'. Could this have been the first glimmerings of the later very popular dressing up as black people by white entertainers who sang bastardised versions of Negro songs? The American Al Jolson introduced us all to talking pictures doing just that, and no BBC programme surpassed in popularity *The Black and White Minstrel Show*, which was completely composed of such, now distasteful, caricature.]

'Between the tobacco smoke, the heated atmosphere, the smell arising from the drink and the foul breaths, and the coarse laughter and yells in the place there was cause enough to daunt the heart of the philanthropist. Before the Free and Easy was put down at the Crown Tavern, I remember of one simple-minded man who was much addicted to getting tipsy, and it was quite a common occurrence for Mrs. N... to make the pretence of taking an extra care over him, which she did by putting her hand in his pockets and taking the greater part of his money. This I had seen often done, as well as the girls, but it was no use speaking, and Mrs. N... continued to rob the man as long as he frequented the tavern.'...

All the three Misses N... were ultimately married, but not to men of any high position in life. Two of them at least were rather addicted to drink, and as a consequence rendered their homes unhappy, while the husband of H..., brought low by whisky, died in an asylum, leaving his wife and three helpless children.

Chapter v

DUNCAN WAS NOW ENTERING upon a new phase in his life, and one which strengthened his character by making him more acquainted with the scriptures.

About this period an anti-Roman Catholic Mission was inaugurated in Edinburgh, under the auspices of the Free Church ...

Duncan regularly attended these meetings night after night...

'The people poured into the Church from all quarters of the city, every seat being occupied. The converts from Roman Catholicism sat together in front of the pulpit, and used the Irish-Gaelic Bible from which they alternately read aloud a verse and translated it into English.

'... (One of the converts was a Roman Catholic preacher who) confessed that his church was not acting according to the scriptures in regard to spiritual matters. After making his confession publicly and renouncing the errors of the Roman Catholic Church, he was excommunicated, and a warning given from St. Patrick's Chapel, Lothian Street, by the priest from the pulpit (which I heard myself), and a very heavy curse pronounced upon any of them who would dare to go and hear the apostate priest, who was proselytising among the true believers of Edinburgh. They would, if they went to hear him, be cursed in walking, in sleeping, in eating and in drinking, in fact cursed in everything they did.

'This converted preacher, however, would have been killed had he not received protection, and as he had no liberty in walking the public streets, he was at length sent to Glasgow. But the Jesuitical system of the Romish Church is far reaching. He had only been some two days in Glasgow when he was set upon and cruelly injured by a Roman Catholic mob, who stoned him and tore his clothes. After recovering somewhat he was conveyed to Amcrica, but even there was found out and subjected to similar treatment, and it is here I have lost trace of him.'...

Mr. N... died of typhoid fever, and Mrs. N... took to imbibing larger quantities of liquor and that more frequently which made her very quarrelsome. The daughter M... married a W... R... who now managed the public house business. Mrs. N... would, while in her drunken fits, when Duncan was at home from the Saturday till the Monday, frequently spend her anger on him, but as Duncan would never give her any reply it only enraged her the more, and she often vowed that if 'that dog would only speak, she would be satisfied!'...

W... R... and his wife had many a drunken scuffle, while both of them ran great danger of losing their lives, as knives were frequently brandished during their quarrels. It was about this period that Duncan left his place at Coltbridge and continued out of regular employment for sixteen months, receiving occasional jobs here and there as he was a member of the journeyman Bakers' House of Call, and very regular in his habits. Having done duty for a Mr. McEwan at Corgatehead, and having given satisfaction through his conscientiousness and punctuality, he was offered a permanent situation there which he gladly accepted. Not feeling at all comfortable at the N...'s he sought out comfortable lodgings and was highly satisfied with his new abode where there was quietness, cleanliness and order...

In 1853 Duncan took an illness which resulted in again changing his views on a subject which every young man has to face, as a rule, sooner or later.

'If I were you, Duncan,' said his friend on one occasion, 'I would make a home for myself as soon as possible. Lodgings are just lodgings at the best, and there is always a chance of your being sent to the Infirmary.'

This caused Duncan to reflect, but as he had never had a sweetheart, he wondered where he would go for a wife. He was now twenty-two years of age,... and he at length cast his thoughts backwards and having fond recollections of a certain Miss J. McK... whom he had known at Coltbridge, but who now resided in the west of Scotland, he at last, although he had not seen her for six years, resolved to ask her hand in marriage, if she was yet free.

He found her out, went and saw her parents, and by his modest and manly behaviour, won their hearts, and that of his future wife also, to whom he was happily married in the month of August 1854.

His wife, by her kindness of heart and generous sympathy with all his schemes and aims in life proved herself a worthy helpmeet, and if Duncan had not made this happy choice at the time he did it is a question if his after successful life would have been as great as it really was.

A few years after his marriage he began reading medical books. He made a lucky purchase of Brooke's *Herbal*, which contained many coloured plates and the uses of the various plants. He then bought another volume – *Dr. Skelton's Medical Adviser*, and was able, by following out the directions contained therein to dispense with the help of a regular practitioner, and after his first baby was born he prescribed in the future for all his family, and always with satisfactory results. The neighbours hearing of his cures, began asking for the same remedies, and by obtaining relief recommended him to the notice of others, so that his circle of patients gradually extended, and he had to make a small charge for the herbs given them, while he still kept up reading all the books in connection with his treatments, that he could lay his hands on. One of the books which stimulated him most to persevere in the course of life he was making out for himself, was the Life of Samuel Thomson of America, who wrought many wonderful cures by simple remedies.

Duncan of course gathered all the herbs he prescribed himself, and as he wrought at his occupation with Mr. McEwan from five am till ten pm, it can easily be imagined that Duncan had now made up his mind to win success, and clung to his purpose with Scottish tenacity and faithfulness.

He was very fortunate in curing a patient after he had been given up by the doctors in the Infirmary as being 'incurable', and past all human skill. Duncan visited him while lying in the Infirmary, and John Aitchison became very anxious that Duncan would take him in hand, and his wife also pressing him anxiously on the same point, that at last, and reluctantly he consented to do what he could for him.

'I endeavoured to get at the first cause of his ailings, as that has always been, with me, one of the most primary importance. After an examination of John I found that his liver, stomach, heart and kidneys were all very much out of order indeed, and so I began with what is known among Botanicals as the Thomsonian System, with the happy result that John began to get better. Being a baker to trade, I advised him to give up all thought of going back to his business, but to look out and try and obtain employment where he would be continually breathing the fresh air. Taking my advice, he made application at the General Post Office for a vacancy

'He received a start as a supernumerary. Shortly after this he was examined by a medical man and pronounced to be 'as sound as a bell, or a rock', and receiving a certificate of perfect health was duly appointed a regular letter carrier. This was in the year 1860, and to this day (1897) still continues on duty in Edinburgh, with a sound and healthy body.'

Many a one came to Duncan for a cure after this as John Aitchison recommended him to all who mentioned their ailing to him.

A man suffering from a severe cold having been made better brought a brother of his to ascertain if any remedy would be of avail for him. 'I did not wish to have anything to do with this case, as I had often seen him lying struggling on the streets, while four, or six men were trying to keep him still, as he was greatly afflicted with St. C [sic] fits. He, Thomas Winter, was about forty years of age. He had been under the best skill in the Infirmary, and was now acting as a porter to do any kind of light work, and had now done so for four years.

'During this period he allowed the physicians to do as they desired with him, but with all the high skill available, he became no better. I obtained his whole history from him, and after many questions, I arrived at the conclusion that the suffering and pain he endured was not caused by those epileptic fits, but the effects of some other derangement, and that a serious one also.

'When I mentioned to him what my opinion was, he did not believe me, far less submit to my treatment. At last he did give in, and between three and four hours after he had taken the medicine, he was relieved of the cause of his suffering, a large tapeworm, measuring sixteen yards long.

'After this he never had another fit, although he sometimes had a slight return of a feeling of falling, but continuing the medicine he at last entirely recovered, and gave up using any more of the remedies.

'I may mention another similar case, that of a young woman. She had been very much troubled with 'falling sickness', as it was called, or severe fits, and had been treated by the medical men for the same, but instead of recovering, gradually grew worse. After hearing how she was affected, I concluded it was a case of tapeworm with this young woman – she was twenty two years of age – and told her mother, who was more than surprised that I should even as much as hint of such a thing being the matter with her daughter.

'She complied, however, to let the daughter try the medicine, with the result that she discharged a whole animal from her bowels, which on measuring I found to be forty-eight feet long with its head.

'The head of the tapeworm is not frequently seen, and when I applied a magnifying glass to it, it bore the appearance of a young serpent. The head had a few inches of a neck attached to it bearing the form also of a serpent's. The young woman completely recovered and is still living and enjoying good health.'

We will only mention one other case before proceeding further. A man, John C who had been sorely distressed with asthma for eleven years was brought by a friend to Duncan. His breathing was very bad, but in two months he was well and free from his distressing complaint.

In thus narrating these cases, it must be distinctly understood that no reflections are cast upon any medical men for their inability to give permanent relief to the patient under his charge, but only to show how successful Duncan was in thus curing what had been deemed hopeless cases.

These cures of course got noised abroad, and Duncan, as the weeks went past, found himself very frequently pressed for time to attend to his baking business and his patients.

In the summer evenings he spent a considerable part of his scant leisure in collecting herbs, and familiarising himself with their various names and medicinal qualities, so that there were few herbs with which he was unacquainted. Blackford Hill and its surroundings, the Queen's Park, and Burntisland in later years, were his favourite haunts for gleaning his useful harvest.

On one occasion while cutting some herbs he needed, a gentleman approached and enquired what he intended doing with the herbs. Duncan without hesitating a moment as to what use his enquirer was going to put his information to, stated his purpose in doing so, and ere he was aware a rain of questions poured in upon him as to the names and uses of the multifarious plants growing near at hand, all of which Duncan was as familiar with, as the faces of his own children.

Having received satisfactory replies, the gentleman then acquainted him with the existence of the Edinburgh Botanical Society, and strongly advised Duncan to attend its weekly meetings.

He did so, and when he made his appearance, he received a very flattering introduction to the members of the Society present for his botanical knowledge from the gentleman who had asked so many questions upon a previous occasion, and who was none other than the worthy President himself!

Duncan was now in his element, and soon put several of the members to shame by the extent of his knowledge of plants. On one occasion, after the President had returned from his holidays, he brought with him specimens which he had collected. One of these he was rather proud of, and began stating its great virtues, and how that it was not to be met with, unless at a considerable distance from Edinburgh. While the President was speaking, Duncan was observed shaking his head, as much as to say there was something wrong. He was rather shy in rising to speak, but at length did so, and to the horror of the members present, actually differed from the learned President! The plant in question was supposed to be a specimen of the Purging Flax. Duncan stated modestly, but firmly that what the President was showing off was not the true flax, but one very much resembling it 'and as for that plant,' said Duncan, 'you might continue drinking away at the infusion from it, but it would never have any influence on the body, whereas a quarter of an ounce of the real Purging Flax would be sufficient for a strong person to take', and in concluding Duncan promised, hastily enough, and on the spur of the moment, to present to the Society on the following week a specimen of the true flax, along with the other herb.

As may be imagined next evening there was a full muster of the members, anxious to ascertain how Duncan would acquit himself. The President had stated that it could not be obtained within a radius of sixteen miles from Edinburgh. On the night of the meeting, Duncan, after leaving duty and going home to tea, went down to a spot called Bells Mills Braes – no more than two miles from the Society's place of meeting, and collecting specimens of each kind, presented them to the gaze of the members, with the result that Duncan carried off the honours of the position, by showing that the President was wrong in the statement he made,

Duncan was one of the most indefatigable collectors of herbs, and every week had specimens brought to the Society for the benefit of the members.

As there was no shop in Edinburgh for the supplying of herbs to the public, and as Duncan saw that there was a necessity, at least in his own case, for such a place, he broached the subject at one of the meetings, with the result that, as none of the members were willing to undertake the responsibility, as they considered the risk too great and likely to prove a failure, he determined to make the venture himself.

He had some difficulty, however, in finding what he considered suitable premises and when he did succeed there was a great reluctance on the part of the agent to let the place for such a purpose.

'To sell herbs! Why, the people in that district are all healthy. There is no use for a shop of that kind. It will likely turn out a failure also, and what will be found in the shop to pay for the rent?'

To show that when physicians have failed to afford relief or affect a cure, and that herbalists have succeeded in many instances we quote the following from Besant's *Life of Edward Henry Palmer*, late Professor of Arabic at Oxford, died 1883.

'It was in the year 1859 that Palmer began to be threatened with symptoms of pulmonary consumption. These rapidly increased, and became at length so alarming that he was sent to one of the best physicians. He was told that his situation was extremely critical and that, in fact... he had better put his house in order, because in a few months at best, he would cease to exist...

'There was at that time a certain herbalist living at Cambridge, named Sheringham... I have been assured by a physician that many of the herbs used by herbalists do actually possess the valuable medicinal properties attributed to them... There are still in fact thousands of people, especially in the great towns, who would not willingly consult any other doctor than the herbalist. The man Sheringham was one of these unlicensed practitioners. Palmer did take his advice and did follow the treatment as commended by him.

'It was simple: it consisted of a single very strong dose of lobelia, a herb which produces, I am told, effects similar to those of hemlock. The patient was first seized with a violent attack of vomiting; then a cold chill laid hold of his feet, and slowly mounted upwards; it froze his limbs, which he could no longer move, and struck his heart, which ceased to beat, and his throat, which ceased to breath. They had sent for a doctor by this time.

' 'I felt myself', he said, describing this experience, 'I felt myself dying; I was being killed by this dreadful cold spreading all over me. I was quite certain that my last moments had arrived. By my bedside stood my aunt, poor soul, crying. I saw the doctor feeling a pulseless wrist, watch in hand; the cold dews of death were on my forehead; the cold hand of death was on my limbs: up to my lips, but no higher, I thought I was actually dead, and could see and hear but not speak, not even when the doctor let my hand fall upon the pillow and said solemnly 'He is gone!'

' 'There was no pain, except the feeling of intense cold', he used to add, nor was he in any concern, except that he wished he had finished a certain book he had begun and he wondered whether in the next world he would have the chance of finishing it...

'And then?'

'Then he recovered. He recovered suddenly. New strength came to him; he not only got the better of this poison, but the lobelia... got the better of his disease. The consumption was arrested, and he was no more troubled for the rest of his life, except on one occasion, with any more anxiety about his lungs. This strange story is absolutely true.'

Duncan offered to pay down an instalment of rent, but all was of no avail, the agent would not let him have the premises. On acquainting his master, however, with the circumstances he called upon the proprietor with the result that Duncan got permission to have the shop, for an herbalist's business.

Affairs however were not yet completely settled. He had to find security for the rent, and not being overburdened with the riches of this world, he was at a loss what to do. The quality of perseverance amid difficulties so inherent in his character, came to his aid, and he resolved to take advantage of Mr. John Hope's kind offer, made to him in past years, that if he required any assistance he was to call and put him in remembrance of it. Duncan did so, and stated the case to his kind benefactor, and the security he required.

Mr. Hope, however, would not become security for the business premises, owing to his having had to pay very heavily for failures in similar instances.

'He said that he could not send me away disheartened, and gave me a sum of money as a present which was far better and of more value to me at that time than merely a security, and so this enabled me to stock my premises and lay past a little for future needs, which was far more that I ever expected. Mr. Hope has been a good friend to me in various ways, and he seemed to know exactly what I most required at that period. May the Lord reward him, as I know mine is not a solitary instance, as he has helped many others in similar ways, and it would fill a volume of a goodly size if his benefactions to the citizens of Edinburgh alone were recorded.'

Duncan opened his shop as an herbalist on the 25th May 1860. He still wrought at his trade, while his wife looked after the shop, but as more customers came when he was behind the counter, he felt that it would be incumbent upon him to give up either the one or the other. His master was very kind to him, and told him if his business failed his place would be open to him.

Duncan accordingly gave up the baking, and devoted his whole time to his duties of a herbalist. His friend Mr. Hope again stood him in good stead in a rather peculiar case which befell him, and gave him a considerable amount of annoyance.

He had bought a quantity of herbs through a traveller from London for which he received a discharged receipt. Being satisfied with the herbs, Duncan gave a second order, for which he also paid. Imagine then his astonishment when, some six months after this last transaction he was, owing to the firm with which he then dealt falling, called upon to forward the sum of sixteen pounds, which the accountants said he was liable for. Duncan wrote back stating the account was paid, and stated he held the discharged receipt.

No notice was taken of this, and when a second demand came asking for payment he began to be troubled and annoyed and more especially when a final notice came stating that if not paid within three days he would be taken to court for its recovery.

Not having a very high opinion of the profession of law and the gentlemen therein engaged, he resolved to take Mr. Hope's advice who advised Duncan, after hearing all particulars and see-ing discharged accounts, not to take any notice of any further communications which came from London, but to send all such to him, and accordingly Duncan was saved an immense amount of future annoyance.

His business, instead of being a failure became more and more extended month by month, and customers failing of relief else-where came from various parts of the country to consult him.

We may here mention a case in which the herbal treatment was very successful after the physicians, many of them being the most eminent men of the profession, having failed to afford relief.

A Miss Gibson who resided with her mother in ... Square, Edinburgh had been ailing for several years. She was only twenty four years of age, but when Duncan first saw her she appeared twenty years older, owing to the pain she suffered, through a severe ulcerated leg on which there were thirty sores all requiring to be separately dressed. Miss Gibson had been recommended to have her leg amputated as the only means of saving her life. Disliking the idea of losing her limb, she was conveyed from

Edinburgh to London, from there to Dublin, then to Glasgow and ultimately back again to her own home. There was but one consensus of opinion by all the medical men, there was no cure but amputation. All this was told to Duncan before he even volunteered to administer any palliatives, and he felt that by undertaking to work a cure by aid of the medicines at his command his would be a difficult task indeed.

The leg was carefully examined, and Duncan undertook to do all in his power for the young woman. It is needless here to state what remedies were applied to the leg and the infusion of herbs taken, but gradually Miss Gibson began to improve. By and by she became able to walk up and down the streets, and she was soon restored completely to health, that is in nine months, not a long period considering she had been under medical treatment for several years.

Not having much of this world's goods, she made Duncan a strange offer. As extra payment for being restored to health and strength she offered to sit in the window of Duncan's place of business and shew off her leg, and tell who cured her after all the physicians she had tried had done their best and failed, but needless to state this strange offer was not accepted!

When this successful cure of an almost hopeless case got noised abroad, as it soon did, it materially added to increase and develop Duncan's business. He had now succeeded so well that he insured his life for two hundred pounds, and having been able to get two of his children into the Heriot schools where they received a free education he felt some of his burdens materially lightened.

During April, May and June Duncan often visited Duddingston Loch where, in the early morning with boots and stockings cast off and trousers rolled up, he waded in the water to procure the various herbs he desired, thus saving expenses. On other occasions he walked to Blackford Hill where he would procure large bundles of needed plants, often weighing one hundredweight, which he carefully conveyed home, where, after tying them up on small bundles, they were hung up to dry, the various smells and scents exuding from them in the process being very pleasing to the olfactory nerves.

Many and many a time he would, having a few minutes to spare, stand perfectly still and make an endeavour to count the numerous rabbits feeding and playing near at hand, frequently fifty in number.

The fresh air of the summer morning, the blue sky overhead, the virgin tint of the trees away down in the valley, the song of the lark and humming of bees made Duncan feel for the time, as if he belonged to another world, and made him relish those morning walks more and more, so full of beauty and reflecting in his heart and soul the peace of heaven itself.

On one occasion while returning from Dysart whither Duncan went once a year to collect certain needed herbs he was returning towards the station carrying his bundle when he came across a gang of men working by the roadside re-laying pipes for the conveyance of gas. The weather was extremely hot and sultry, and several of the workmen had thrown off most of their upper garments. One of them, just while Duncan was passing, threw his cap off his head at him, which missed him, and landed at the other side of the road, while he cried out 'To h... with you, man and take that cap with you!' By a sudden impulse Duncan stood still and cried out so as to be heard by all 'I can't take your cap for I'm not going that road!'

West Wemyss, Burntisland and Aberdour were also places where Duncan collected...

At this point in the manuscript sixteen sheets have been cut out of the book. What appears to be the last eight have been loosely re-inserted. We cannot know now by whom this was done, when or why. It seems that at least some of the missing pages described the illness of Duncan's first child, John, and of Duncan's fight against the compulsory vaccination against smallpox, a fight in which he showed as much determination as he did in his constant battles against drink and what he always called popery. The book resumes:

... desiring the presence of his brothers and sisters gave ... them all a few parting words, among his last words being 'If you are all converted I will meet you in heaven again.' Further on he mentioned a bright light which he seemed to perceive, but by this time he was blind. His mother said 'Oh, John, that will be the angels coming for you!' This he seemed to realise and in a short time afterwards passed quietly away.

This son John was ten years when he died, and on the day he was buried his younger brother Duncan took ill also and died, the disease being very severe.

Two of the girls of the family turned ill, but the smallpox being of the ordinary type they soon recovered.

Duncan's patients of course soon suffered by his absence in attending to his own children. Several of them died, but the devastation was general all over the city, but Duncan passed safely through this trying time without the epidemic touching him or his wife.

'I could relate many awful cases which occurred during this time. The cry was raised against all those who would not comply with the compulsory law, to compel them to have their children vaccinated, or re-vaccinated, because the majority of people were like sheep following a great superstition. Eyes had they but they saw not, ears had they but they did not hear. This compulsion I would never comply with, but I resisted it with all my strength. As I have seen several hundreds of cases, and deaths resulting from the poisoning of the blood through vaccination, I am strongly of opinion that every child which escapes disease from this lymph suffers in some form or other. Lymph used to be called, and rightly, 'corruption', and it is still the same – a blood poisoner.

'A bad case of blood poisoning through vaccination comes to my memory. A family of the name of Grant who lived in Middleton's Entry were all vaccinated by Professor Sir James Simpson, since deceased. For eight years the eldest son was a mass of sores from his back down to his heels. He was told by his medical adviser if spared till he reached the age of twenty-one, he might then be free from the loathsome eruption, nice consolation truly, and a splendid testimony also to the benefits (!) resulting from vaccination!

'A brother of Mrs. Grant's was also taken very ill after being vaccinated by the same Professor, and with the same lymph. This man became a policeman, and nine years after he had been operated upon and with such success the epidemic I have referred to broke out. This man was chosen by the Medical Officer of Health for the city to go with him on his rounds and to help him in reporting all cases of small pox.

'This duty Mr. Thompson successfully fulfilled for some time. One day, however, he failed in appearing at his post. A messenger was sent to see what had gone wrong, who returned with the answer that he had been attacked with small pox. Dr. L... accordingly called upon him, and said he after he had seen him, 'I'll have him admitted to the hospital.' His wife pleaded for him to be left where he was. She was quite willing and ready to send away her seven children out of the house if only her husband was allowed to be left at home. In vain. Her pleadings were useless. In a quarter of an hour a cab containing three men drove up her door, and while one man held the wife, the others carried him away by force.

'When his sister Mrs. Grant heard of this high-handed proceeding, she called at the hospital and enquired for him. This she did regularly for three weeks, and although she was not allowed to see him, she always got the answer that he was doing nicely and improving. Imagine then her grief and astonishment when, on enquiring as usual, she was told by one of the nurses that her brother was lying in the dead-house awaiting interment!

'His body was soon laid in the grave. We pass over the grief caused by his death. And more to my point, showing to what lengths medical men will go to uphold the rite of vaccination. Thompson had his life insured in a London society and was registered on their books as vaccinated. A strange thing now happened. When the certificate of death was forwarded to the society it read that the patient died of small pox and was unvaccinated. The Society thereupon refused to pay the amount of insurance, as they considered the deceased had dealt unfairly with them.

'Even although 'vaccination was to be saved from reproach', by such base methods, the friends of Thompson disliked such practices and took the case to law with the result that the former certificate had to be abrogated and then the money was paid, and the medical man who signed the false certificate – Thompson being vaccinated twice – was exposed.

'It is only those who have studied both sides of this great question who perceive that the law as it stands sins against God and against man. I am one of those who have seen some of the alarmingly evil results which take place immediately after the innocent children have been blood poisoned. My twenty years experience convinced me of the wickedness of this compulsory blood poisoning, and I chose rather to suffer the penalty that the law inflicted, rather then submit to having any more of my children vaccinated, and run the terrible risk of this death, or ill health, as a material consequence, for to my certain knowledge some hundreds of children have been killed through this vile operation.

'The first time I was brought before the Court for refusing to blood poison my child, I was determined to lie in prison rather than pay the penalty, and did not take even a copper in my pocket. The sentence was thirty five shillings (including expenses) or ten days imprisonment.

'The officers recording me stated what I had to pay, but I mentioned that I had no money with me and had no intention of paying. Whereupon I was conveyed downstairs into an empty cell, there to await the arrival of the van to convey me to Calton Jail. However, while waiting there, I heard my name, in a short time afterwards, called out. I answered to the call, when the officer said 'Your fine is paid so you are at liberty to go.' I believed what he said, although I did not know who paid my fine, and walked out a free man once more.

'Six months afterwards I was summoned to appear again, and in the interval a very severe case had happened which I will relate.

'In Thomas Street, Leith Walk, there resided a man named... He had a child, perfectly healthy, just a gem of a baby, whom he did not like to get vaccinated, as he disbelieved in blood poisoning for the counteracting of a disease which might never come upon the baby. He was, however, too poor to pay the fine in case of refusal and could not afford to lie in jail. The child was vaccinated accordingly by Dr. Husband. In three days afterwards inflammatory appearances set in, which gradually went down and arms and over the...

[This is the end of the pages cut out of the manuscript book, and at this point we return to the book itself.]

...whole body of the child who showed symptoms of suffering great pain. In about eight days the parents could hardly bear to look upon the their own child, as it was all broken out in ulcerous holes, while its eyes were nearly falling out of their sockets to appearance, and it could not see. Death came however as a true friend and mercifully relieved it of its sufferings.

'The minister and missionary and likewise the neighbours testified to the child being one of the nicest babies that any one would desire to possess until the period that it was vaccinated.

'The day before the child died the father called upon me to ascertain what should done. I advised him to go and lay the charge of death upon the doctor who vaccinated the child.

'The medical man sent a substitute, but the child had just died before he arrived. Intimation of death, however, was sent to him. The case was taken to court, and the father stated that the child had been poisoned. The case was remitted to the Medical Officer of Health to deal with, and as the child had died on Friday it was buried the day after owing to the number of children in the house.

'After a great many preliminaries the body of the child was exhumed and examined. Week after week past and no word was received by the father even though he called repeatedly at the proper quarter until finally he received the reply 'Oh, yes, your child died – from natural causes!'

'The doctor who poisoned the child was mentioned by name be me in court and the circumstances of the case narrated, but I was duly fined for refusing to allow my healthy child to run the risk of being similarly dealt with.'

[This is the end of Duncan's manuscript. Several sheets at the back of the book are left unused.]

A Nineteenth Century Herbalist's Casebook

(With comments on the treatments used by Dee Atkinson, a twenty-first century herbalist.)

AMONGST THE DOCUMENTS left by Duncan Napier was a long hand-written paper describing some of the cases he treated. It was not really a casebook, for it describes only spectacular successes, and even Duncan must have had some failures. Nor, unfortunately, does it give much information about the treatments and medicines he used. Its great interest is in showing the variety and severity of some of the cases an Edinburgh herbalist was called upon to treat in those days.

Although there is no way of knowing whether it was ever sent to him, the document was in the form of a letter to his son, also Duncan Scott Napier, then a soldier somewhere in the dreadful fields of France during the First World War.

The first few pages of the document have been omitted. They are merely a brief account of how Duncan came to be a herbalist. He wrote of that in much greater detail in his autobiography, reproduced as Appendix Three of this book.

I think it is valuable to reconstruct, so far as possible, the treatments Duncan used in the cases he describes. Dee Atkinson, herbalist at Napiers today, has done this, and her contribution to this section is given in each case after Duncan's description of it. Fortunately, some of Duncan's old recipe books are still in the possession of the Napier family. Well-worn and battered, and liberally bespattered with unknown liquids, these are still legible, and Dee has consulted them in trying to reconstruct Duncan's treatments.

TO MY DEAR SON DUNCAN SCOTT NAPIER

What is contained in this Book is a short account, first of how I was led to take an interest in the study of Herbalism, Medicine, and Plants. Especially their use in Healing session. And second a brief account of some of the more outstanding cases of which I was successful in treating both before and after the start of my Herbal Business. I have thought that this record might be interesting to you, and to your Posterity after you, and the work of compiling it was done during the dark nights of the great European War and specifically the winter of 1917-18, when you were fighting in the War in Flanders.

During the months of April and May I used to get up very early in the morning to get my herbs, and I might have been seen standing in Duddingston Loch any time in the morning from four to seven o'clock, with my shoes and stockings off and trousers rolled up as far as they would go, pulling up Buckbean. It was as much as I could do in those cold mornings to stand in the cold water, but as I usually carried home a heavy bag full of Buckbean, well up for a hundredweight, I got a good heat before I got home. It took me two days before I got each load tied in bunches and hung up to dry.

Then I would go out to Blackford Hill where I got Mullein, Agrimony and Greater Comfrey, and if it was past five in the morning when I reached the hill I was rather late, and so had to cut the herbs with all speed. If I had a few spare minutes when the bag was filled I would take a stroll over the hill, and that was of course long years before it was ever thought of securing the hill for Edinburgh. Then, in those quiet summer mornings I would stand still for a few minutes and see how many rabbits I would count, and it was not unusual for me to count fifty.

Another district which I visited near to Edinburgh was Corstorphine Hill, where I got raspberry leaves, and Mother of Thyme.

I also used to go further afield, and crossed the water to Burntisland, where in the Bind woods, the quarry and other places in that vicinity I gathered Agrimony, Mountain Flax, Bloodroot, Cranesbill, from the last mentioned of which was made the Anti-Cholera Powder. On one occasion a man with a double-barrelled gun and two dogs came upon me in the Bind Woods and suspecting me for a poacher, demanded to see what I had in my bag. I threw out the contents on the ground from which he saw that I had no rabbits. I feared that he would not even let me take the herbs, but I packed them in again, talking all the time: I was, however, cleared off.

After leaving the woods I looked over a fence into a field where men were working. A conversation began between myself and the farmer who was there, and as he seemed interested, I told him my business and of my expulsion from the Bind. He then took me up onto a hill and showed me what of the surrounding country was his, and told me that I had perfect liberty to go into all the woods and fields on condition that I did not steal his corn. I thereafter called this part my big garden in Fife.

I took a journey once a year to Dysart where I always got a large quantity of Agrimony and Centaury.

Occasionally I went to Ratho by train and walked from there to Kirkliston where I got Yarrow and always a good supply of Raspberry leaves. Rasps. are in abundance there, and when I was having a feast of them I was always reminded of the woods of Penicuik and of the days when I was young.

One year, when visiting Uncle Alan in Fifeshire, I saw great clumps of splendid Mountain Flax. This was somewhere in the direction of Donnibristle and at the time when the miners were out of work. I suggested to one or two of them that they might gather some Mountain Flax for me. A week or two afterwards they came with a huge sackful of the finest Flax I had ever seen. I paid them one shilling per pound for it, but was at a loss to know what to do with so much of it. I thought of selling some of it in London, but ultimately I kept it, and every bit of it was used up, and it paid me well.

John Aitchison

This was a friend of mine who was also a baker, and lived opposite me in the Grassmarket. His wife's Father who lived with them was an old sailor who lost his leg in battle, and in those days a plaster of boiling pitch was put on the stump to stop the bleeding. This old sailor professed to cure Jaundice in an hour, and the mixture was a bottle of ale and a pennyworth of powdered alum. The ale was brought to the boil and the alum dissolved in it, the whole costing sixpence. That patient was charged five shillings, the dose being administered in the house, and the cure being successful before he was able to leave the house.

Now John fell into ill-health and was unable for his work and I tried to get the Botanical Society to help me in taking up his case, but they refused, and there was nothing else for him to do but to go into the old Infirmary.

He was there for some months but he got worse. By his wife's request I visited him several times, and one time found him very much alarmed as several in the same ward had died. He would not let me away until I promised to attend him when he came out. The doctor's statement was that his heart, liver and stomach were so deranged that he would never recover, so on his dismissal card was 'Incurable.'

I made some herbal mixtures and treated him for some time and he seemed cured so he applied for some work in the Post Office. He was thoroughly examined and tested by Professor Dunsmure who pronounced him to be 'as sound as a rock.'

He carried postbags from the Post Office to the outskirts of Morningside for 33 years. By this time, owing to age and failing health he had to retire, and he received from the Post Office officials not only a pension, but thinking they had not given him enough for his long service, they gave him a double pension to keep him and his wife comfortable. His friends gave him an easy chair, a timepiece and handsome ornaments.

One gentleman to whom John had delivered letters for a number of years sent a paragraph to *The Scotsman* giving him a very high character and summing up the distance of miles he had travelled – some thousands of miles.

John was feeling very proud of this notice, and also grateful to me for having cured him so many years before, so in recompense he got a pamphlet printed telling about his cure and for several days my friend Sergeant Ross and myself distributed those bills to the small villages of Causewayside and Comiston, and on the way some such remarks as these were heard: 'He must be a grand doctor that when he employs a gentleman like that, in regimentals, to deliver bills!'

First Case of Tape Worm

This happened in the days before I opened my shop, when I was always reading and finding out about herbs and making up various mixtures. I had often seen this man going about the streets, and I had also seen him lying on the ground in one of his epileptic fits, it taking six men to hold him down.

He was a big strong healthy-looking man about 36, and he was known to take those fits frequently. He had been a patient in the old Infirmary for years, and for several years he had been a porter in the old Infirmary. The doctors had tried all sorts of experiments on him, such as making issues for matter to run round his neck and over his head, indeed all sorts of operations were tried, but nothing was of any avail, and he was even allowed to drink as much whisky as he could before going to bed, but nothing seemed to cure those fits, or 'Falling Sickness', as the doctors called it.

[NOTE: 'Issues' were drains, usually silk threads, inserted under the skin, or into an artificially induced ulcer, with the belief that any 'bad matter' would be drained away.]

His brother called at my house and asked if I could do anything for him, but it could not be wondered if I hesitated long before agreeing to try such a notorious case. However, his brother was so urgent that I reluctantly said I would do what I could. The man himself came to see me one day, and I had a long conversation with him, trying to get at the bottom of his trouble. After listening to his story and hearing all his symptoms I concluded that those fits were caused by Tape Worm. I agreed to try on condition that he would pay the cost of getting some ingredients sent from London.

In due time they arrived and it took me some days before the mixture was ready. About the second day after he had taken the medicine a large worm came away, one large unbroken piece measuring 16 yards long, as well as several smaller pieces, and from that day he never again fell.

Some time would elapse and the old symptoms would return, showing that the draining of the system was still there, he could not speak but would come flying up to my shop which was by that time open, and a dose of skullcap would speedily restore him.

Herbs have always been used to treat cases of worms, and patients still come for consultations looking for natural remedies. Worms have a habit of re-occurring and treatments often need to be repeated. Duncan Napier would repeat his worming dose after two weeks to make sure that he had completely got rid of the worms.

One of his tapeworm formulae was based upon Fluid Extract of Male Fern, together with Extract of Butternut and Glycerine. The Mail Fern Extract was one of the most popular vermifuges, and was especially efficient against tapeworms, which it both kills and expels. It was widely used by vets, as well as by herbalists. This was a well-balanced formula, with the butternut acting as a bowel tonic with a gentle purgative action, and itself having a distinct action as a worming agent. Glycerine was often used as a mild laxative. It has a sweet taste that would have made this bitter medicine more palatable.

Duncan Napier's tapeworm patient, who was also an epileptic, would have benefited from the scullcap, which has traditionally been used in epilepsy. The herbs contained in that formula would have calmed him down and acted as an anti-spasmodic, which would have reduced the incidence of his fits.

Napiers Scullcap Compound was used for all types of spasm and nervous weakness, and was often used to ease cramping bowel problems. Many of the compound medicines had a number of uses and were the backbone of the herbal practice. Scullcap Compound is still made to the original recipe and I find it invaluable in treating chronic fatigue and post-viral problems.

A Baker's Eczema

In the days before I opened a shop I knew a baker who was very ill with eczema. This was a long-standing case and both arms were badly affected, and I had no feeling to begin, but he persuaded me to try something on him. He took the medicine for a few weeks, but as there was not much improvement he became down-hearted and sarcastically remarked to me 'I suppose I will have to drink a tubful before I am cured. If you were like other drug people your dose would be in drops.' I said that I could give him medicine in drops if he would like it, but he said he did not believe I could, and he would like to see it. I produced a quarter of a tea-spoonful of something and asked him just to taste it, never dreaming that he would swallow it all at a gulp.

My wife and I thought he was choked, for he could not speak for some seconds, and the water gushed from his eyes, nose and mouth. His first word when he was able to speak, and uttered with a great oath, was what did I call that. On my saying 'I call that Number Six,' he replied with another oath that he would not like to taste my Number Twelve. He did not come back to me for a month and during that time had gone to some man who called himself a Skin Professor. This man professed to cure him, saying that he was the only man who could do it. So accordingly he paid down £5 for his course of medicines and expected to be perfectly cured.

But when he had finished the medicine he was disappointed to find that he was no better. He again called on the Professor who said to him 'But that was only the first course you had, and you will require several and each course will cost £5.'

He said he was not prepared to pay any more at the time but would return, but this he never did.

About a month after this he came again to me, and said he was quite prepared to resume the former treatment if I would agree to it. He continued for about three months and by that time he was pretty clear, and my cure only cost him sixpence a week. That was indeed just a slight difference from the £5 courses that would-be Professor was ready to extort.

Co-bittersweet powder was taken internally and ointment (The General's) outside.

[NOTE: There is no record we can find of what the General's Ointment was, nor where it got its name.]

The old recipe for
Bittersweet Powder Compound is:

3oz Pulverised Queens Delight
4 oz Pulverised Blue Flag
3 oz Pulverised Sassafras Bark
3 oz Pulverised Uva Ursi
7 oz Pulverised American Mandrake
6 oz Pulverised Pareira Brava
6 oz Pulverised Liquorice Root
6 oz Pulverised Bittersweet
9 oz Pulverised Senna Folia
6 oz Pulverised Yellow Dock Root
6 oz Pulverised Guiacum
6 oz Pulverised English Rhubarb
6 oz Pulverised Ginger
4 oz Pulverised Burdock Root
4 oz Pulverised Bogbean
5 oz Pulverised Figwort

This complicated recipe is a fair example of the sort of formulation favoured by an earlier generation of herbalists. Today, the tendency is towards using much simpler mixtures, with only three or four ingredients.

Herbs and roots were brought into Napiers in both cut and powdered form. Compound powder mixes, such as the Bittersweet, were packed into small grease-proof envelopes that contained a single dose. This was taken by mixing the powder in water, and usually ended up as a suspension rather than a solution.

The basis of formulae such as the Bittersweet Compound were

bowel tonics and laxatives. Senna, rhubarb and liquorice encouraged the bowel to function regularly. Constipation results in a toxic build up in the system and leads to toxins coming out in the skin and causing eruptions such as the baker's eczema.

Yellow dock, figwort and blue flag all support the action of the liver, helping to cleanse and detoxify. Liquorice has an anti-inflammatory action, and was often used in skin problems

This formula would have had a very bitter taste, enhanced by the action of the bittersweet. The bitter taste encourages the body to release digestive juices, liver enzymes and bile, thereby encouraging digestion.

The theory went that poor digestion led to leaky gut syndrome, allowing substances to leak out of the gut and set up allergic reactions.

Napiers had a lot of success in treating skin problems, and was often able to help where other treatments had failed. I have been honoured in inheriting this wealth of knowledge and have been able to work with some of Duncan Napier's formulae.

Eczema is a problem that is on the increase, and more sufferers are turning back to the traditional methods of treatment. Whilst I usually make up a formula specifically for the individual, I still make up and use some of Napiers stock medicines. The Bittersweet Compound gradually fell out of favour, as some of the original herbs in the formula were no longer used. Mandrake in particular was withdrawn from internal use due to worries about its safety. Napiers best known skin formula was the Blood Purifying Tonic, which become one of the ten best sellers.

Ointments for eczema and skin problems were more widely used than creams, and were particularly popular when the sufferer had a trade that involved coming into contact with potential allergens, such as flour. My feeling is that today the baker would have been given Napiers Marigold Ointment, which is still made. Ointments sit on the skin and provide a protective layer, allowing the skin to heal underneath.

Today our best-selling skin product is a cream, Starflower Cream. I have based it on some of the Napiers ideas of using anti-inflammatory and healing herbs, and on some of the often forgotten traditional skin healers such as chickweed.

Mr. Burt

He had been ill for several months, was gasping for breath and for weeks had been sitting on a chair and could not lie down in bed. On a certain day the doctors said they could do no more for him, and that he would certainly be dead that night by 11 o'clock.

His wife was in a great state and was advised to come to me and ask if I could do anything to save him. I called in the evening and seeing he was so far gone, I consented to do what I could for him, only on the condition that he would take my medicine only, and that he would not be interfered with by the doctors.

Consent was given and I told them to make preparations for a vapour bath and left them, promising to return later on. On my returning I gave him the Thomsonian course of medicine, then the vapour bath.

After perspiration he was sponged with vinegar and water, nearly cold, rubbed dry and put into bed and given a vomit. He was afraid to lie down in bed in case he would choke, but he was persuaded and I left him.

When I called next forenoon, I was pleased to see him breathing freely, having had a good sleep, and now looking like a new man. I continued treating him with suitable medicine and within two months he was quite well and returned to his work as a reader in Ballantyne's Printing Works.

He kept well and was able to attend his work for about nine months. Unfortunately, one very cold day he went to Duddingston Loch to see the skaters, although he had been warned to be very careful and not expose himself to cold. His wife, happening to call on me that Saturday afternoon and mentioning where he had gone to, I knew what would be the result and advised his wife to hurry home and be prepared for her husband being brought home as he would not be able to walk, and this was what actually happened, for he was brought home in a cab.

I treated him for seven days but without success. Two doctors were then called in, but he died, and they tried their best to prove that I had poisoned the man, and such news spread quickly!

On the funeral day the Registrar came hurrying round to me

for the Doctors would not fill up the Certificate and the people were all waiting. Of course the thing was quite simple. I filled it up as I had been attending him last. Dr. Littlejohn then sent down to me demanding to know all the ingredients of the medicine the man had last taken, his two officials bringing with them all them all the bottles and boxes (nearly 100 in all) for me to identify. The bottles had contained Anti-Spasmodic Tincture – now called Skullcap – but I refused to give any information as I had no intention of giving away my secret remedies. The Doctors tried all in their power to prove a case of manslaughter, but failed.

On a number of occasions Duncan Napier was at loggerheads with the powers-that-be over his herbal medicine. Whilst his treatments were thought of as almost heroic and his reputation was huge amongst the people of Edinburgh and its environs, he was sometimes a thorn in the side of the authorities. Trips to the doctor were expensive and sometimes the treatments were worse than the disease. Mercury, antimony and calomel commonly appeared as medicines, and hospital was a last resort.

Napiers provided a gentle and much cheaper alternative. Duncan Napier was a disciple of the American herbalist Samuel Thomson, and sometimes used his vapour baths and steaming herbal treatments on his patients. Heat raised the body's core temperature, making it an unfavourable climate for bacteria and viruses. Sweating allowed the body to rid itself of toxins. It also helped to relax the lung tissue, allowing the patient to breathe more easily.

The medicine that Duncan gave to Mr. Burt was his Scullcap Compound. The earlier formula for this medicine contained Lobelia Herb and had an anti-spasmodic action on the lungs as well as relaxing the whole body.

Scullcap Compound Formula, 1865

Pulverised Capsicum
Pulverised Skunk Cabbage
Crushed Valerian root

Pulverised Black Cohosh
Pulverised Cramp bark
Crushed Oregon grape
Crushed Bayberry
Golden seal root
Lobelia herb
Scullcap herb.

These herbs were all added to a percolator and allowed to steep in a hot water and alcohol solution for a number of days before the tap was opened at the base of the percolator and the mixture allowed to drip through.

Two Brothers from Leith

A certain Mr. Ward was first a patient in the old Infirmary for ulcerations in the throat and afterwards an out-patient. He had several operations on his throat by some method of burning and suffered so tremendously that one day he said to the three doctors who were present that he could stand no more, and if they attempted to burn his throat again he would knock them down. And as they persisted, he was as good as his word, and knocked the three men down to the floor one after the other, and then fled out of the building.

As he passed through the gate the keeper advised him to come to me, and he entered my shop in a terrible state, scarcely able to speak and pointing to his throat, which was in a sad way, the flesh being quite burned away to the bone. I took him in hand, gave him something soothing and healing and in time he was cured.

Some time after, this man's younger brother, who was an apprentice to a skinner at Water of Leith, took inflammation in one of his knees (caused by standing in water washing skins), and was taken to Chalmer's Hospital.

In the ward with him were other three men with the same complaint, and one after another died after their operation. This young man was so terrified for his turn coming that he sent for his brother to come and see him. When his brother came he asked him to come close as he had something to tell him. On his brother bending down to him, he clasped his arms round his neck and held him like a vice, and said nothing would make him leave hold and that his brother must take him home with him. So he had to get a blanket twisted round him, carry him out and take him home in a cab.

Then the brother came up to me to me and told me all the particulars and I gave him something to apply. In about a week or so he was brought up to me in a cab for me to examine; in about a fortnight after he managed to walk up with the help of two sticks, and then in about another week he could walk with one stick, and by and by in a few weeks time he could walk up alone and was quite cured without the need of amputation. As he was a bound apprentice he was being compelled to return to his work, but as I had warned him that to stand in the water again as he had done would prove fatal for him, his Masters listened to his petition and he was released. He ultimately went to Glasgow and became apprentice to a house painter.

A year or two afterwards he visited me and on my asking him about his knee, he laughingly said that he thought the leg that had been cured was the stronger of the two.

Inflammatory joint problems were common in Mr. Napier's clinic. The conditions that people worked in were far from ideal, and health and safety at work was not a concept. Women especially suffered from 'housemaid's knee', from long hours spent scrubbing floors and blackening the range. Liniments were popular and Napiers Stimulating Liniment was made up in a pestle and mortar and contained cayenne, turmeric, sassafras and turpentine. These herbs, especially the cayenne, would have acted as a rubefacient, encouraging blood supply to the area and thereby helping to reduce the inflammation.

Turmeric was also made into a tincture and given with herbs such as willow bark, bogbean, guaicum and feverfew to treat joint inflammation. I use similar prescriptions in clinic, and often combine my own formula with some of the Napiers stock remedies.

Herbalists such as Napiers had their own repertoire of standard medicines that they sold across the counter. These were formulae used to treat the most common complaints of the time – cough syrups, cold and flu mixes and indigestion remedies. Years of empirical knowledge and research had gone into these recipes and they were closely guarded secrets. Patients who needed to see the herbalist had prescriptions made up specifically for them. These would often contain blends of the stock formulas and some single tinctures. One of Duncan Napier's prescriptions for a patient who consulted him may have contained as many as 40 different herbs

Duncan was an 'Eclectic' and was well versed in the different schools of herbal medicine. He read widely and was aware of herbalists such as Thompson as well as the works of Gerard and Culpeper. He was also one of the last, and one of the best, of the old time artisan herbalists, who had no formal training, but knew from experience which herbs produced the required effect, and had no hesitation about prescribing them.

Miss Gibson

This woman had a very sore ulcerated leg from knee to toe, and when I saw her, her leg had no form, and she herself looked like 40, although she was only 24. A friend who was a member of the Society tried to get the Society interested in her case and to help her, but they could not see their way to do this.

Some kind ladies sent her to Ireland, Glasgow and London, but all doctors agreed in saying that nothing short of amputation would cure her, and to this she would not submit.

I treated her with purifying medicine, but as she was poor and the quantity of Slippery Elm she would require was too costly, the treatment by simple fomentations was slow and tedious. She lived in St. James Street, and of course was quite unable to walk the distance to the shop, but in due time she was cured and could walk alright.

She was so grateful after recovery that she offered to sit in my window and exhibit herself as a cure, and tell all how her leg was saved, but needless to say her kind offer was not accepted. It was certainly a wonderful cure, for the leg was so bad that I hesitated long before doing anything.

> Napiers Blood Purifier was one of the mainstays of the practice and is still made to the original formulation today. Ulcers, boils and scrofulous skin eruptions all benefited from the Blood Purifier. It contains burdock, yellow dock, oats, red clover, Napiers Scullcap Compound and a Compound infusion of Calumba. The resulting liquid contains over twenty herbs. Time and time again in clinic I find myself coming back to the original Napiers formula. Herbs have a synergistic effect, and the action of a combination of herbs is often more than the sum of the action of the individual herbs, and this is certainly the case with these formulae. Often when patients have bad acne, and we have tried a range of herbs, I find myself using the Blood Purifier and finding it successful.

No Imitations

On a shelf in my shop window might have been seen bottles containing Tape Worms, with the dates and length of each. Some from children from two years of age – the length being seven feet. I remember one day a group of a doctor and six students standing round the windows and the Doctor explaining those bottles and their contents to his students and expatiating largely on them as such splendid imitations – Oh, the irony – as if I had need of imitations when I had the real thing.

Two Children Cured of Dropsy

The father of these children, and also their Uncle, called on me and pled me to come and see these children who were fast dying. On calling, I found them very ill indeed, their faces as well as their bodies swollen and about blind.

The Doctor attending them said he would be back next morning to operate on them if they were still alive. One of their relatives came back with me to the shop – then my first shop – and I gave him some medicine for them.

In the morning the Father came to tell me of the happy result, that the children were sitting up in bed, wonderfully cheery and asking for their breakfast. When the Doctor called in the forenoon he simply held up his hands in amazement saying what a blessing he had not come earlier – it must have been evident to him what effect an operation would have had on those dying children.

And in about two weeks time they were perfectly cured.

About a year or so afterwards the boy took a severe chill and was nearly suffocated through acute bronchitis. A messenger was sent to the Father's shop to come at once and bring a Doctor. He came to me and begged me to come with him and treat his boy.

Before entering the bedroom the Mother cried out 'Have you brought a Doctor with you?' and her husband replied 'I have brought Mr. Napier', and the Mother cried out 'Confound you, why have you not brought a proper Doctor with you?'

On hearing these words I felt that I was not wanted and was preparing to go, but this the Father would not listen to, but reminded the Mother how I had cured both of the children, and she ultimately complied and said 'If you think you can do anything come forward and try.'

On seeing the gasping condition of the boy I gave him a vomit of Lobelia, and when he had vomited freely, his mother asked him how he felt, he said, 'Mother, I am all right now. I am cured.' Thus I earned the gratitude of the Mother.

If Duncan Napier was correct in his diagnosis of these two sick children, they both had heart problems. Dropsy was the name given to a severe form of fluid retention that was caused by heart problems. It would be unlikely to find two cases of this in two small children of the same family, unless it involved some sort of viral attack on the heart muscle.

However, heart medications were often prescribed by herbalists, and one of their best known heart medicines, foxglove, has been taken over by the orthodox profession and synthesised to give us the prescription drug Digoxin. Duncan was well used to using foxglove, and he had a formula for a tincture combination that included scullcap and cherry bark. Nowadays herbalists use lily of the valley for heart problems. Under the 1968 Medicines Act, the use of lily of the valley is restricted to herbal practitioners who are operating under the terms of the Act.

Story of a Decayed Jawbone

This was a serious case of a young woman who had been under great doctors for a long time with her top jawbone in a decaying state. She was recommended by someone to visit at my shop, but when I saw her sore disfigured face swollen to double its size, I was afraid it was too far gone to cure.

However, she besought me so that I said I would try, knowing full well myself that although my treatment might not be able to cure her, it could do her no harm. I gave her some special herbs to steam her face sometimes, as well as applying large Slippery Elm poultices. I persuaded her to continue this treatment and when fully a month had passed, part of the bone began to protrude, and I was afraid that worse might follow, and so it did, for one day she brought me a bit, about half of the jaw bone, which had come away with actually four teeth in it.

It was a sad sight, but still I thought the Slippery Elm would do its good work along with some inward treatment. The swelling gradually subsided and in several months time a new jawbone began to grow, and as the months passed teeth began to appear also.

When the bone came out it left a great scar in her face, but by degrees it became perfectly natural like. I told this story to a certain Doctor who laughed at it unbelievingly, but I gave him the address of this lady so that he could call and see for himself, as she had kept the bone and could show it to him, but whether he went or not I do not know, which is really a small matter. But what I really know is that she often came to my shop and thanked me heartily for the wonderful cure I had performed, and also that her face was in no way disfigured, at least not more then by a slight scar.

This happened amongst the early years in my first shop, and gave me more confidence than ever in the wonderful healing properties of the Herbs. The lady of this story afterwards married and had a fine family.

This is one of the strangest and most unlikely of stories. Some years ago at a herbal conference I was relaying this story to an audience of fellow practitioners and students. When the laughter had died down, our guest speaker for the evening, a well known Herbal Vet., told a story of one of the animals that he had treated, a dog, that had re-grown part of its jaw bone following an infection in the bone.

My own maternal grandfather lost all his teeth at the age of thirty-eight. At the age of forty, he began to produce new teeth, and by the age of forty-five had a full set of perfectly sound teeth which lasted well until his death forty years later. Such apparent contradictions of the supposedly immutable laws of nature are indeed rare, but not unknown.

We rarely see such acute patients in our clinics, but in Duncan's time the use of slippery elm poultices to draw out infection was common practice, even on seemingly hopeless cases.

Story of a Bald Head

A poor woman came to see me one day with no hair on her head and asked me what I could do for her. Her system was low down, and thus her hair had come out until she looked as if her head been shaved. I gave her both outward and inward treatment and by the time three months had passed her hair not only had begun to spring but had a good strong growth. By this time of course she thought she was quite cured and I did not see her for about a year.

One day when she came, lo, all her hair had come out again and she was quite bald. Well, she had the same remedies again, and stuck well into them, and in time her hair actually grew in a second time, even a stronger growth than the first.

This is a story that will strike a chord with many practitioners. Patients often feel that as soon as their symptoms are removed, they are cured. Herbal medicine aims to get down to the root cause of a problem, and help the body to re-establish a healthy pattern. Often the outward visual symptoms such as hair loss are an indication of a deeper, more long term problem. Our body regards our hair and nails as disposable. If our body is under stress, or poorly nourished, our hair and nails can stop growing, or even fall out. Duncan recognised this with his patient, and he will have treated her with herbs and diet to strengthen her system, at the same time as using one of his famous hair tonics.

Napiers Eucalyptus Hair Restorer was famous beyond the Scottish border; it was a popular seller through Napiers growing mail order business. We still make the hair restorer, faithfully following Duncan's recipe. It involves using large quantities of eucalyptus, sage, rosemary and southernwood, heating them in a big covered boiler and allowing it to cool. The smell from the release of the volatile oils while this is being made is strong enough to clear any blocked sinus!

Ulcerated Legs

A certain man called at my shop and was very anxious for me to come and see a friend of his. I called and saw a very disturbing case of a woman who was sitting in front of her bed with her legs hanging over, and those legs were terribly swollen and ulcerated.

She could not lie down in bed, and had been in this painful condition for several months. Her legs required a good deal of steamings and fomenting, and we also persuaded her to lie down in bed. Sometime later I returned to give her a lot of internal warming medicine.

I attended her for about six weeks and left her able to go about the house. The man who asked me to attend her was really no special friend, but having heard of her state took pity on her and thought he could have her cured. She was deeply grateful to him and also to myself for the wonderful cure. And this man after seeing this wonderful cure, sent me many more patients

Leg ulcers are still a common problems, and many patients who suffer from circulation problems have swollen legs. The skin becomes tight and irritated. Patients are often given a mild steroid cream to apply and this leads to thinning of the skin. The thin skin breaks easily and an ulcer forms. Every time I see a patient with hot, tight swollen calves, I know we have to take immediate action.

Strengthening the blood vessels and improving the circulation is the long term objective, but this will take months of treatment to effect. Whilst this is happening there is still a need to protect the skin. Poke root ointment was developed by Duncan for just such a purpose and is still the best product.

To make Poke Root Ointment, marigold, red clover, comfrey and poke root herb are bound together in a piece of muslin and suspended in a pot containing a blend of simmering oils and waxes. The hot oils and waxes extract the active ingredients from the herbs, and after forty-eight hours the ointment can be poured. Sadly, the ancient tradition of ointment making has all but died away. Herbalists used to have a range of ointments that they used, and their use was often multi-purpose. Napiers made Marigold, Arnica and Golden Seal Ointments. I have seen Poke Root Ointment being used on the cracked teats of cows in the milking parlour, and, from the same jar, used for rough skin on the farmer's feet, showing clearly the multi-purpose value of that ointment.

A Wart Removed

A well-known Colonel had four sons who were doctors and they were urgent in their appeals to their Father to go to the Infirmary and have this wart cut off – but he was nervous about it and could not make up his mind to go.

This wart which was growing on his neck, under his ear, was about half an inch long, and was the largest developed wart I had ever seen. I gave him Co. Tincture of Sanginarian [sic] which he used for a few weeks. He was very anxious that I should cure it, first to show to his sons what I could do, but after a few weeks he was afraid it was not going to come off, but I thought it showed signs of shrivelling up and growing less, and advised him to continue.

His sons continued worrying him to go to the Infirmary, but he did not wish to go, and stuck well into the stuff for a few weeks longer, not wanting to be beat. So one day after washing himself and drying his neck he seemed to feel the wart had disappeared, and lo, it was in the towel. It had come off beautifully, leaving scarcely a mark behind, and his four doctor sons were surprised to say the least of it, for they had never seen anything worked like that before.

> *Sanguinaria canadensis*, or blood root as it is commonly known, was used as a paint for warts and verrucas. It has an ability to shrink tissue, and to treat inflammation topically. A snuff of blood root was used to treat nasal polyps. Duncan usually treated warts with a combination of internal medicines and blood root paint. Warts are viral in origin and Napiers Blood Purifying Tonic and Echinacea Tincture make a perfect combination. The echinacea supports the immune system, helping the body to tackle the virus and the Blood Purifying Tonic, with its burdock and yellow dock, supports the liver.

Toothache Cured on the Spot

Late one Saturday evening a gentleman and his son opened my shop door and asked if I could pull a tooth. I said 'No, but I can cure toothache.' 'Nonsense, Nonsense' he replied and went off in a passion.

About twenty minutes later they both returned and remarked 'You said you could cure toothache'. 'Yes', I said, 'but you did not seem to believe me.' 'If you can cure toothache have sympathy for myself and my son.

I then said 'I will cure it in four minutes.' I applied some of the powder on to the tooth and told the boy to keep his mouth shut the while I kept talking to the Father. By and by I asked 'What about the toothache?' 'Oh, the pain was all gone.'

Then the Father asked my charge – a penny, only a penny. He was very grateful for the cure, and he must have recommended it often, for many a penny box did I sell.

This powder was composed of powdered alum and table salt, mixed with one part Spanish Pellitory. Wet a piece of wadding, dip it in the powder and put direct into the tooth.

Duncan's early toothache powder, made from powdered herbs, table salt and alum, was refined by John Napier and a tincture version was produced. A wad of cloth or cotton wool was soaked in the tincture and it was held in the mouth over the painful tooth. The herbs helped to anaesthetise the area and dealt with any gum inflammation. If the tooth was rotten it would still need to be pulled out. In the islands of Scotland, and in some of the poorer mainland areas it was not uncommon for people to have all their teeth pulled out, often as a 21st birthday present! This eliminated the need of ever having to consult a dentist for tooth problems. I was reminded of this when attending an elderly patient who came from the Outer Hebrides. She commented loudly to her grandson, that I was 'a nice girl, with a fine set of teeth'. Obviously a desirable attribute!

Tape Worm Mixture

The Right Honourable Neil Dow was told by Doctor Kirk about my wonderful Tape Worm medicine, so he took a good few bottles with him when he returned to America, and gave them to friends who found it gave every satisfaction.

He praised this mixture in the American papers in the State of Maine, and one morning there were heaps of letters for me enclosing a dollar and asking to have a bottle sent to them – one bottle containing one dose was sufficient for a cure.

General Marshall

He had been 40 years out in India and now he was home and had been ill for eight years with Eczema. I knew his maid Maggie Spence, and I had known her parents at Dalry Mills, or Dry Mills as it was called.

This maid was in attendance on the General and I fancy she was getting tired nursing him and washing the cloths. One day she happened to say to Mrs. Marshall if the General knew her Doctor he would soon be cured.

Mrs. Marshall repeated this to her husband about the Edinburgh herbalist and Maggie sent a note to me asking if I would call some day. I wrote to her saying that I did not care to come unless invited by the General himself – this invitation I had by return.

Then I went out to his house at Millerhill and when I saw the General he gave me a searching look and asked if I was Mr. Napier the Herbalist. On replying that I was he asked if I could do anything for him, but I said I would have to examine him first.

After I had examined him, his first question was what I called his disease, and when I said 'Chronic Eczema' he seemed satisfied as that was the same version as the Doctors. His body was covered from head to foot with white blisters and was a very bad form of wet eczema and on my saying I could cure him on one condition, he was naturally anxious to know what that condition was.

'Well,' I said, 'I must have a free hand. You must take my medicine only and none of the Doctor's and indeed the Doctor must not interfere with me in any way.' He was quick with his actions and quickly called for writing materials and wrote two Post Cards to the Professor and family Doctor asking them not to call in the meantime.

Then he asked me when I would begin and I said 'As soon as I returned,' and also said 'Seeing the Doctors had been trying to cure him for eight years I would be glad if he would allow me as many months', and so the compact was sealed.

I gave him inward medicine to purify his blood and the Poke (Root) Ointment for outward application. I visited him at Newton

House Millerhill twice a week and persevered with him and the treatments, and even before the eight months expired he was cured and my farewell visit left him with a skin perfectly pure from head to toe.

Time rolled on and I heard nothing of them for ... when suddenly one Sabbath day a messenger appeared on horseback at my house, telling me that the General was seriously ill and begging me to come out and see him. I had the greatest difficulty in getting a cab, but ultimately I succeeded.

On seeing the General and hearing his condition my heart sank, for I saw it was hopeless. He was suffering from acute inflammation of the liver and had been ill for a few weeks: Ah, if only they had sent for me sooner, but now it was too late. But I did all I could for him and stayed all night with him, and the next day it was with great sorrow that I had to say to his wife and family that I could do no more for him and that he would not last long, and he died in a few days.

After informing the Doctor that he was dead, the Doctor refused to give his certificate of death and they were greatly put about. The eldest son rode in to me on horseback in great haste, asking what they should do. I told him that I could fill it up as I was the last in attendance.

Unfortunately he had not the certificate with him and had to return for it post haste and I filled it up in proper order and signed it.

Of course the Professor who had been in attendance before me could have signed it if he had been inclined. It was a very large funeral and not knowing anyone I waited for the Minister and sat beside him.

After the service the butlers brought wine of all kinds. The Minister refused the wine, saying he never took any, and of course I refused also, and so it passed on, and there were very few who had the hardihood to oppose the splendid example that the Minister had set, and the General was buried in the Grange.

Duncan, like other herbalists of his time, was used to visiting his patients at home, and he often had to work around the doctors and physicians who were already attending the patient. There was a lot of competition for patients, and a lot of suspicion on both sides. Many people came to the herbalist as a last resort, and when they found that the treatment worked, they started using the herbalist as their main health care practitioner. When I started practising at Napiers many of my patients had been consulting John Napier for years, and were firm believers in plant medicine and a naturopathic approach to health.

Nowadays many people use the herbal clinics at Napiers as their first port of call for any of their health problems. We now run specialist clinics for skin problems, menopause, arthritis, mother and baby as well as the popular low income clinic. Herbal medicine is enjoying a popular revival, with moves being made to regulate the sale of herbs and to create a register of recognised qualified herbalists. I am confident that we will see what was once an age-old divide between doctor and herbalist vanish altogether, and herbal medicine will become part of a national health care system.

Index

Some other books published by **LUATH** PRESS

LUATH GUIDES TO SCOTLAND

The North West Highlands: Roads to the Isles
Tom Atkinson
ISBN 0 946487 54 5 PB £4.95

Mull and Iona: Highways and Byways
Peter Macnab
ISBN 0 946487 58 8 PB £4.95

The Northern Highlands: The Empty Lands
Tom Atkinson
ISBN 0 946487 55 3 PB £4.95

The West Highlands: The Lonely Lands
Tom Atkinson
ISBN 0 946487 56 1 PB £4.95

South West Scotland
Tom Atkinson
ISBN 0 946487 04 9 PB £4.95

POETRY

Poems to be read aloud
Collected and introduced by Tom Atkinson
ISBN 0 946487 00 6 PB £5.00

Scots Poems to be Read Aloud
Collectit an wi an innin by
Stuart McHardy
ISBN 0 946487 81 2 PB £5.00

Bad Ass Raindrop
Kokumo Rocks
ISBN 1 84282 018 4 PB £6.99

Bad Ass Raindrop
Kokumo Rocks
ISBN 1 84282 018 4 PB £6.99

Sex, Death & Football
Alistair Findlay
ISBN 1 84282 022 2 PB £6.99

Men and Beasts: wild men & tame animals
Val Gillies & Rebecca Marr
ISBN 0 946487 92 8 PB £15.00

Madame Fife's Farewell and Other Poems
Gerry Cambridge
ISBN 1 84282 005 2 PB £8.99

Picking Brambles and Other Poems
Des Dillon
ISBN 1 84282 021 4 PB £6.99

Kate o Shanter's Tale and Other Poems
Matthew Fitt
ISBN 1 84282 025 1 PB £6.99

Luath Burns Companion
John Cairney
ISBN 1 84282 000 1 PB £10.00

Immortal Memories (of Robert Burns)
Selected and edited by John Cairney
ISBN 1 84282 009 5 HB £20.00

THE QUEST FOR

The Quest for Arthur
Stuart McHardy
ISBN 1 84282 012 5 HB £16.99

The Quest for the Celtic Key
Karen Ralls-MacLeod and
Ian Robertson
ISBN 1 84282 031 1 PB £8.99

The Quest for the Nine Maidens
Stuart McHardy
ISBN 0 946487 66 9 HB £16.99

The Quest for the Original Horse Whisperers
Russell Lyon
ISBN 1 84282 020 6 HB £16.99

FOLKLORE

Scotland: Myth, Legend and Folklore
Stuart McHardy
ISBN 0 946487 69 3 PB £7.99

The Supernatural Highlands
Francis Thompson
ISBN 0 946487 31 6 PB £8.99

Luath Storyteller: Highland Myths & Legends
George W. Macpherson
ISBN 1 84282 003 6 PB £5.00

Tales from the North Coast
Alan Temperley
ISBN 0 946487 18 9 PB £8.99

POLITICS & CURRENT ISSUES

Scotlands of the Mind
Angus Calder
ISBN 1 84282 008 7 PB £9.99

Trident on Trial: the case for people's disarmament
Angie Zelter
ISBN 1 84282 004 4 PB £9.99

Uncomfortably Numb: A Prison Requiem
Maureen Maguire
ISBN 1 84282 001 X PB £8.99

Scotland: Land & Power – Agenda for Land Reform
Andy Wightman
ISBN 0 946487 70 7 PB £5.00

Old Scotland New Scotland
Jeff Fallow
ISBN 0 946487 40 5 PB £6.99

Some Assembly Required: Scottish Parliament
David Shepherd
ISBN 0 946487 84 7 PB £7.99

Notes from the North
Emma Wood
ISBN 0 946487 46 4 PB £8.99

VIEWPOINTS

Scotlands of the Future: sustainability in a small nation
Eurig Scandrett (ed.)
ISBN 1 84282 035 4 PB £7.99

Eurovision or American Dream? Britain, the Euro and the future of Europe
David Purdy
ISBN 1 84282 036 2 PB £3.99

NATURAL WORLD

The Hydro Boys: pioneers of renewable energy
Emma Wood
ISBN 1 84282 016 8 HB £16.99

Wild Scotland
James McCarthy
ISBN 0 946487 37 5 PB £7.50

Wild Lives: Otters – On the Swirl of the Tide
Bridget MacCaskill
ISBN 0 946487 67 7 PB £9.99

Wild Lives: Foxes – The Blood is Wild
Bridget MacCaskill
ISBN 0 946487 71 5 PB £9.99

Scotland – Land & People: An Inhabited Solitude
James McCarthy
ISBN 0 946487 57 X PB £7.99

The Highland Geology Trail
John L Roberts
ISBN 0 946487 36 7 PB £4.99

'Nothing but Heather!'
Gerry Cambridge
ISBN 0 946487 49 9 PB £15.00

Red Sky at Night
John Barrington
ISBN 0 946487 60 X PB £8.99

Listen to the Trees
Don MacCaskill
ISBN 0 946487 65 0 PB £9.99

ISLANDS

The Islands that Roofed the World: Easdale, Belnahua, Luing & Seil:
Mary Withall
ISBN 0 946487 76 6 PB £4.99

Rum: Nature's Island
Magnus Magnusson
ISBN 0 946487 32 4 PB £7.95

TRAVEL & LEISURE

Die Kleine Schottlandfibel [Scotland Guide in German]
Hans-Walter Arends
ISBN 0 946487 89 8 PB £8.99

Let's Explore Berwick upon Tweed
Anne Bruce English
ISBN 1 84282 029 X PB £4.99

Let's Explore Edinburgh Old Town
Anne Bruce English
ISBN 0 946487 98 7 PB £4.99

Edinburgh's Historic Mile
Duncan Priddle
ISBN 0 946487 97 9 PB £2.99

Pilgrims in the Rough: St Andrews beyond the 19th hole
Michael Tobert
ISBN 0 946487 74 X PB £7.99

FOOD & DRINK

The Whisky Muse: Scotch whisky in poem & song
various, ed. Robin Laing
ISBN 0 946487 95 2 PB £12.99

First Foods Fast: how to prepare good simple meals for your baby
Lara Boyd
ISBN 1 84282 002 8 PB £4.99

Edinburgh and Leith Pub Guide
Stuart McHardy
ISBN 0 946487 80 4 PB £4.95

WALK WITH LUATH

Mountain Outlaw
Ian R. Mitchell
ISBN 1 84282 027 3 PB £6.50

Skye 360: walking the coastline of Skye
Andrew Dempster
ISBN 0 946487 85 5 PB £8.99

Walks in the Cairngorms
Ernest Cross
ISBN 0 946487 09 X PB £4.95

Short Walks in the Cairngorms
Ernest Cross
ISBN 0 946487 23 5 PB £4.95

The Joy of Hillwalking
Ralph Storer
ISBN 0 946487 28 6 PB £7.50

Scotland's Mountains before the Mountaineers
Ian R Mitchell
ISBN 0 946487 39 1 PB £9.99

Mountain Days & Bothy Nights
Dave Brown and Ian R Mitchell
ISBN 0 946487 15 4 PB £7.50

SPORT

Ski & Snowboard Scotland
Hilary Parke
ISBN 0 946487 35 9 PB £6.99

Over the Top with the Tartan Army
Andy McArthur
ISBN 0 946487 45 6 PB £7.99

BIOGRAPHY

The Last Lighthouse
Sharma Krauskopf
ISBN 0 946487 96 0 PB £7.99

Tobermory Teuchter
Peter Macnab
ISBN 0 946487 41 3 PB £7.99

Bare Feet & Tackety Boots
Archie Cameron
ISBN 0 946487 17 0 PB £7.95

Come Dungeons Dark
John Taylor Caldwell
ISBN 0 946487 19 7 PB £6.95

HISTORY

Civil Warrior [Montrose]
Robin Bell
ISBN 1 84282 013 3 HB £10.99

A Passion for Scotland
David R Ross
ISBN 1 84282 019 2 PB £5.99

Reportage Scotland
Louise Yeoman
ISBN 0 946487 61 8 PB £9.99

Blind Harry's Wallace
Hamilton of Gilbert-
field [intro/ed Elspeth King]
ISBN 0 946487 33 2 PB £8.99

Plaids and Bandanas: from Highland Drover to Wild West Cowboy
Rob Gibson
ISBN 0 946487 88 X PB £7.99

SOCIAL HISTORY

Pumpherston: the story of a shale oil village
Sybil Cavanagh
ISBN 1 84282 011 7 HB £17.99
ISBN 1 84282 015 X PB £7.99

Shale Voices
Alistair Findlay
ISBN 0 946487 78 2 HB £17.99
ISBN 0 946487 63 4 PB £10.99

A Word for Scotland
Jack Campbell
ISBN 0 946487 48 0 PB £12.99

ON THE TRAIL OF

On the Trail of William Wallace
David R Ross
ISBN 0 946487 47 2 PB £7.99

On the Trail of Robert the Bruce
David R Ross
ISBN 0 946487 52 9 PB £7.99

On the Trail of Mary Queen of Scots
J Keith Cheetham
ISBN 0 946487 50 2 PB £7.99

On the Trail of Bonnie Prince Charlie
David R Ross
ISBN 0 946487 68 5 PB £7.99

On the Trail of Robert Burns
John Cairney
ISBN 0 946487 51 0 PB £7.99

On the Trail of John Muir
Cherry Good
ISBN 0 946487 62 6 PB £7.99

On the Trail of Queen Victoria in the Highlands
Ian R Mitchell
ISBN 0 946487 79 0 PB £7.99

On the Trail of Robert Service
G Wallace Lockhart
ISBN 0 946487 24 3 PB £7.99

On the Trail of the Pilgrim Fathers
J Keith Cheetham
ISBN 0 946487 83 9 PB £7.99

On the Trail of John Wesley
J Keith Cheetham
ISBN 1 84282 023 0 PB £7.99

GENEALOGY

Scottish Roots: step-by-step guide for ancestor hunters
Alwyn James
ISBN 1 84282 007 9 PB £9.99

WEDDINGS, MUSIC AND DANCE

The Scottish Wedding Book
G Wallace Lockhart
ISBN 1 94282 010 9 PB £12.99

Fiddles and Folk
G Wallace Lockhart
ISBN 0 946487 38 3 PB £7.95

Highland Balls and Village Halls
G Wallace Lockhart
ISBN 0 946487 12 X PB £6.95

CARTOONS

Broomie Law
Cinders McLeod
ISBN 0 946487 99 5 PB £4.00

FICTION

Driftnet
Lin Anderson
ISBN 1 84282 034 6 PB £9.99

The Road Dance
John MacKay
ISBN 1 84282 024 9 PB £9.99

Milk Treading
Nick Smith
ISBN 1 84282 037 0 PB £6.99

The Strange Case of RL Stevenson
Richard Woodhead
ISBN 0 946487 86 3 HB £16.99

But n Ben A-Go-Go
Matthew Fitt
ISBN 1 84282 014 1 PB £6.99
ISBN 0 946487 82 0 HB £10.99

Grave Robbers
Robin Mitchell
ISBN 0 946487 72 3 PB £7.99

The Bannockburn Years
William Scott
ISBN 0 946487 34 0 PB £7.95

The Great Melnikov
Hugh MacLachlan
ISBN 0 946487 42 1 PB £7.95

LANGUAGE

Luath Scots Language Learner [Book]
L Colin Wilson
ISBN 0 946487 91 X PB £9.99

Luath Scots Language Learner [Double Audio CD Set]
L Colin Wilson
ISBN 1 84282 026 5 CD £16.99

Luath Press Limited

committed to publishing well written books worth reading

LUATH PRESS takes its name from Robert Burns, whose little collie Luath (*Gael.*, swift or nimble) tripped up Jean Armour at a wedding and gave him the chance to speak to the woman who was to be his wife and the abiding love of his life. Burns called one of *The Twa Dogs* Luath after Cuchullin's hunting dog in *Ossian's Fingal*. Luath Press was established in 1981 in the heart of Burns country, and is now based a few steps up the road from Burns' first lodgings on Edinburgh's Royal Mile. Luath offers you distinctive writing with a hint of unexpected pleasures.

Most bookshops in the UK, the US, Canada, Australia, New Zealand and parts of Europe either carry our books in stock or can order them for you. To order direct from us, please send a £sterling cheque, postal order, international money order or your credit card details (number, address of cardholder and expiry date) to us at the address below. Please add post and packing as follows: UK – £1.00 per delivery address; overseas surface mail – £2.50 per delivery address; overseas airmail – £3.50 for the first book to each delivery address, plus £1.00 for each additional book by airmail to the same address. If your order is a gift, we will happily enclose your card or message at no extra charge.

Luath Press Limited
543/2 Castlehill
The Royal Mile
Edinburgh EH1 2ND
Scotland
Telephone: 0131 225 4326 (24 hours)
Fax: 0131 225 4324
email: gavin.macdougall@luath.co.uk
Website: www.luath.co.uk

ANTIFAT PILLS

Dose: Two Pills, three times daily after meals.

Formula: Ext. Fucus ½ gr.
Ext. Glycers ½ gr.

D. NAPIER & SONS
17 & 18 Bristo Place
EDINBURGH, 1

NAPIERS' COMPOSITION ESSENCE

Has been used for over seventy-five years in treating the COMMON COLD and INFLUENZA. Taken at the first sign of trouble, it almost invariably checks it; and it may be used freely by old and young.

The Essence is a powerful stimulant on the circulation, strengthening the whole system, always acting through the stomach.

For cold in the head, catarrh, influenza, hoarseness, chill from exposure and so on, it is unequalled. For bucking coughs, it may be used as a gargle, and ten drops may be taken on sugar. It is excellent for cold night sweats, cramp and cold in stomach and bowels.

Price (including Tax) ...

(vertical side text) PREPARED ONLY BY D. NAPIER & SONS 17 and 18 Bristo Place, EDINBURGH

NAPIERS' BRISTO RUBBING LINIMENT

For relief of Rheumatism, Sciatica, Lumbago, Neuralgia, Headaches: and as a speedy, effective treatment for strains, sprains, bruises, injuries, nerve and muscular aches and pains of every kind.

DIRECTIONS FOR USING.—Rub the Liniment gently but thoroughly into the painful parts. Repeat every four or six hours as may be required.

Must NOT be used if the skin is broken or unsound.

Compounded from: Oil. Camph. Liq. R. Oil. Terebinth. Rect. 5, Oil. Cajuput 5, Capsi. Fruct. 5, Ammon. Carb. 5, Chloroform 7.5, Camphor 25, Meth. Sulicyl. 25, Spt. Vin. Meth. (Indust.) to produce 80.

PL 0896/5017

D. NAPIER & SONS
17 & 18 BRISTO PLACE
EDINBURGH, 1

NAPIERS' S OINTMENT

Rub into the parts with the finger, night, morning, or thrice daily, 1, 2 or 3 times daily.

Prepared from—Calendula, Sambucus, Fofolium Alkanet, Ungus Fulv. ana 1 in each. 25, Spermacet 75, Acid Sulphuric 5, Adeps 10, Sapon. ruh. 15, Paraff. dur. 75, Paraff. Mol. 25, Ol. Rapis. 50.

D. NAPIER & SONS
British & Foreign Medical Botanists
17/18 BRISTO PLACE
EDINBURGH

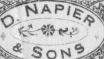

Napiers' HAND LOTION
NON-GREASY

PREVENTS ROUGHNESS AND CHAPPING

RUBBED IN A LITTLE AT NIGHT OR EACH TIME AFTER WASHING

D. NAPIER & SONS
BRISTO PL., EDINBURGH

NAPIERS' HERBAL COMPOSITION POWDER

For colds, chills, and influenza

Dose.—One rounded teaspoonful with sugar. Place the dose in a teacup, fill with boiling water and stir thoroughly. When the contents settle, drink the clear liquid. May be used freely by old and young. May be taken 3 or 4 times daily—More if required.

Active Ingredient.— Each rounded teaspoonful contains approx.
Bayberry 0.9 g; Ginger 0.4 g; Pleurisy 0.4 g; Cinnamon 0.2 g; Cloves 0.1 g.

KEEP MEDICINES OUT OF REACH OF CHILDREN
PL 0896/7043

D. NAPIER & SONS
17-18 Bristo Place, EDINBURGH

PL 0896/5007

NAPIERS' HERBAL BASED OINTMENT
Yellow Pine

To Draw And Soothe
Especially beneficial for boils and minor sores

Directions:—Spread on white lint, press gently into the sore and cover lightly. Repeat 3 or 5 times daily.

Active Ingredients:— Pix. Burgund. 5%;
Pulv. Res. Alb. 1.5%; Alum ol. 1.5%

Keep Medicines out of reach of Children

D. NAPIER & SONS
17/18 BRISTO PLACE
EDINBURGH

Napiers' LOBELIA HERB SYRUP

for
COUGHS
CHEST COLDS
ASTHMA
BRONCHITIS
WHOOPING COUGH

Suitable for
Children and Adults

NAPIERS' LOBELIA SYRUP

For coughs, bronchial asthma and infections of the upper respiratory tract.

KEEP MEDICINES OUT OF REACH OF CHILDREN

SHAKE THE BOTTLE
PL 0896/5014

D. NAPIER & SONS
17/18 Bristo Place,
Edinburgh.

NAPIERS' Herbal Tonic

Especially beneficial when taken after influenza, or in cases of stress and debility after much stress and exhaustion.

Active Ingredients—Each ½ oz contains—Tinct. Scutellaria BHP 0.1 ml; Tinct. Symphoricarpus BHP 0.062 ml; Tinct. Valerian BPC 1949 0.025 ml; Tinct. Viburnum. Op. BHP 0.007 ml; Tinct. Capsicum BPC 1949 0.012 ml; Liq. Ext. Unifa BPC 1949 0.1 ml; Liq. Ext. Damiana BPC 1934 0.1 ml; Liq. Ext. Saive BPC 1934 0.05 ml; Liq. Ext. Humulus BHP 0.062 ml; Liq. Ext. Passiflora BHP 0.075 ml; Liq. Ext. Valerian 0.037 ml; Liq. Ext. Avena BHP 0.037 ml; Conc. Inf. Calumba BP 1948 0.075 ml; Conc. Inf. Gentian BP 1973 0.05 ml.

KEEP MEDICINES OUT OF REACH OF CHILDREN
SHAKE THE BOTTLE
PL 0896/5017

D. NAPIER & SONS
17/18 Bristo Place, EDINBURGH

NAPIERS' HERBAL POWDER
COMPOUND MEADOWSWEET

This powder has a purifying action which helps the elimination of waste matter by maintaining urinary flow.

Dose.—A rounded teaspoonful. Place the dose in a teacup, fill with boiling water and mix thoroughly. Drink the clear liquid when cold. Take two doses daily, the first after breakfast, the second at bedtime. A dose may be prepared at night so as to be ready for the morning. Each dose should be made separately.

Active Ingredients.—Each rounded teaspoonful contains approx.:—
Meadowsweet 0.3 g; Celery 0.3 g; Pellitory 0.3 g; Uva. Ursi 0.3 g; Ginger 0.2 g; Wild Carrot 0.3 g; Bryogo 0.2 g; Burho 0.1 g; Brown 0.3 g; Blue Flag 0.1 g; Cinnamon 0.1 g; Liquorice 0.15 g.

KEEP MEDICINES OUT OF REACH OF CHILDREN
PL 0896/7042

D. NAPIER & SONS
17/18 Bristo Place, EDINBURGH

PL 0896/2006
NAPIERS' HERBAL OINTMENT
CALENDULA

To soothe Wounds and Open Sores.
Directions—Apply on white lint, or rub in gently but thoroughly before or retiring. Repeat 2 or 3 times daily.

Active Ingredients—Extract of Olivus
Fulv. 5; Calendula 5; Symphytum 5; Trifol. 25 in Spermaceti 75. Paraff. Mol. 16; Adeps 1; Cinnamon 5; Sapon Wax 75; Paraff. dur. 75; Sapon. Rub. 10; Oil.

Keep Medicines out of reach of Children

D. NAPIER & SONS
17/18 BRISTO PLACE
EDINBURGH

Established 1860

D. NAPIER & SON.
Botanists.
Consulting Herbalists,
Collectors of British Herbs,
Foreign Herbalists.

17, BRISTO PLACE
EDINBURGH

Medicines

Folio. No.

Agents for D'Nichols (of London)
Publications & Sanitary Productions.

NAPIERS' COMPOUND LOBELIA HERB SYRUP

OPERATIONS.—Expectorant, Relaxant, Diaphoretic, Anti-asthmatic.

USE.—This Lobelia Syrup has been used for up to two-eighty years, with the most happiest results, for the most happy results, with the most happy results in coughs, colds, asthma and infections of the upper respiratory tract. It is an excellent remedy for most affections of the chest.

DIRECTIONS—Adults; one or two teaspoonfuls two or three times daily, at bedtime and throughout the day. It remains special watch to reducing the inflammation of the bronchial tubes. For warm and visceral reach, it gives much soothing relief. For CHILDREN a teaspoonful two or three times daily.

PREPARED ONLY BY D. NAPIER & SONS, Botanic Drughts, 17-18 Bristo Place, EDINBURGH. ESTAB. 1860

Price (including Tax) 1/4.

Napiers'
MYRRH & BORAX
TOOTH POWDER

D. NAPIER & SONS
17/18 Bristo Place
EDINBURGH, 1

DIURETIC ESSENCE

FOR

Pains in the Back, Loins, and Kidneys, Obstruction of the Urine, Inflammation, Dropsy, Gravel, Diseases of the Bladder, and Affections of the Renal Organs.

Dose.—Adults, a dessert-spoonful four times daily. Children from one to two tea-spoonfuls three times daily.

Price 1/1½ per Bottle.

PREPARED BY
D. NAPIER & SON,
BOTANIC DRUGGISTS,
21 Bristo Street, EDINBURGH.

Lavender Flowers
D. NAPIER & SONS · BRISTO · EDINBURGH

NAPIERS' EUCALYPTUS HAIR CONDITIONER
FOR DARK HAIR

A non-oily application for use where the hair has lost its brilliance. Helps to prevent dandruff and stimulate the scalp.

Directions—Apply regularly night and morning, rubbing gently but firmly into the roots of the hair and then the fingers. Allow to dry then brush lightly.

Active Ingredient—Aq. Ext. Eucalyptus 5%; Salvia 6% 3%; Rosemary 8%; Arnica 8%; Camph. 0.1%.

KEEP MEDICINES OUT OF REACH OF CHILDREN
SHAKE THE BOTTLE
PL 0896/5059

D. NAPIER & SONS
17/18 BRISTO PLACE, Edinburgh

PURE SLIPPERY ELM BARK
FOR INWARD USE

This is the inner bark, finely powdered, of Ulmus Fulva of North America. Its use is indicated in cases of mucous inflamation and ulceration of stomach, bowels and bladder; in gastric and duodenal ulcers, diarrhoea, and dysentry; in Bronchitis and Colitis. It soothes, heals and counteracts acidity, and may be given when great exhaustion and debility are present.

DIRECTIONS.—Mix one teaspoonful of the Powdered Bark with the same quantity of sugar, add a little cold water and stir into a thin paste. Add a teacupful of hot milk, slowly stirring all the time. Flavour with nutmeg or cinnamon, and drink warm. This may be prepared with water only using neither milk nor sugar and may be taken twice or thrice daily.

SOLD BY
D. NAPIER & SONS
British and Foreign Medical Botanists
17-18 Bristo Place, EDINBURGH, 1

Napiers'
KIDNEY PILLS
DOSE.

Two pills at bedtime, or One twice or thrice daily.

Each pill contains—Aloes Barb. 1 gr.; Pot. Nit. 1 gr.; Capsicum 1 gr.; Ext. Buchu ½ gr.; Ext. Uvae Ursi ½ gr.; Turps. Venet ½ gr.; Podophyllin 1/16 gr.; P. Buchu and Ol. Junip. q.s.

D. NAPIER & SONS
BRITISH AND FOREIGN MEDICAL BOTANISTS
17-18 Bristo Place, EDINBURGH, 1